CW00546479

HOW TO TREAT ROOT CAUSES OF DISEASE

A Clinical Nutritionist's Guide to Getting Well Again

Gaynor J Greber

Gaynor J Greber
www.gjgbionutrition.org

Cover/images

istock.com
Terry Robinson Technical Author

Proofreader/Editing

Bridget Gevaux
www.abcproofreading.co.uk

Typesetting

aSys Publishing (www.asys-publishing.co.uk)

ISBN: 978-3-9525704-9-4
Alphorn Press

'Listen to your patient, he is telling you the diagnosis'.

'A good physician treats the disease, a great physician treats the patient who has the disease'.

Sir William Osler 1849–1919

Canadian physician and Regius Professor of Medicine at Oxford University 1905–1919

About the Author

Gaynor Greber qualified with excellence from The Institute for Optimum Nutrition in London in 1993.

As a Clinical Nutritionist and Functional Medicine Practitioner, she spent twenty-two years in private practice in the UK before moving to Switzerland.

She is a former member of the British Association for Applied Nutrition and Nutritional Therapy (BANT), and the Complementary and Natural Healthcare Council.

She attended training with The Institute for Functional Medicine and is a former Associate of The Royal Society of Medicine.

Other health books by Gaynor Greber:

Chronic Digestive Disorders–Regaining Health with the Functional Medicine Approach.

On Guard – Build Resilience – Boost Immunity – Beat Infection.

Contents

INTRODUCTION

Do you feel frustrated with life and desperate to experience good health again?

Are you constantly struggling with illness despite being on medication designed to treat your symptoms?

Do you often seek and try new dietary approaches based on hearsay, or follow recommendations you have read about somewhere but feel it is futile as you are not making progress?

Do you—despite all attempts—continue to feel unwell?

Then this book has been written specifically with you in mind.

If the above scenario sounds familiar, then seeing a functional medicine practitioner or nutritional therapist to guide you through the process of reversing disease and healing your body—focusing on you as an individual rather than just your symptoms—will be the best way forward for you to regain health.

The body is continuously evolving, so you can build a new you at any time in your life—given the right conditions.

Whatever diagnosis you have been given, unless the underlying root causes of your symptoms are addressed at the cellular level, you cannot fully heal.

1

These considerable root causes can range from faulty diet or lifestyle factors—to immune, liver, or digestive dysfunction. I am not talking about disease here, but dysfunction—and there is a huge difference.

Functional medicine is concerned with supporting optimum healthy function in all body systems. This approach uses laboratory test procedures to identify deficiencies, excesses, or biochemical imbalances in body systems. Drug-free, individually designed treatment protocols offer a personalised approach to achieving good health.

Nutrition should be thought of as nature's medicine. Food as calories satisfies hunger pangs, but food contains the nutrients that nourish our bodies and is the 'fuel' for all metabolic function. Every cell in the human body is fundamentally made of nutrients, and your dietary choices determine whether your body receives an adequate, regular supply of the dozens of nutrients required to keep you in good health.

Any symptoms of ill health will always involve either nutritional deficiencies, excesses, or biochemic imbalance within the body systems.

If you are already suffering with illness, it is never too late to take action to reverse chronic disease and restore health. Treating the root causes of your health problems, instead of taking medication for symptoms only, will bring positive results. You will experience remarkable benefits as you journey along this route, sometimes sooner than expected.

I have spent many enriched and absorbing years treating ill health with the functional medicine approach. In recent years, I have been practising and writing health books in Switzerland.

Having gained valuable knowledge attending conferences, workshops, seminars, and meeting wonderful inspirational people and leading authorities in the field of nutrition along the way, I would now like to pass on some of this knowledge.

I continue to be fascinated by both nutritional and functional medicine, and the proven fact that healing foods and supplementary nutrients in doses way beyond the basic recommended levels that prevent deficiency diseases, can prevent, heal, and reverse disease.

As a practitioner, I have witnessed numerous full recoveries over the years in chronically sick individuals, most having spent years on medication, and seeking my help to follow my personally designed protocols only as a final resort.

How often have I heard the words, 'If only I had known earlier'. I believe functional and nutritional medicine should be available options to everyone seeking medical advice, and I am happy to see in recent years that many UK GPs are adding this modality to their practices.

Privately, I practise exactly what I preach. I can guarantee you that eating the healthiest organic, well-balanced, colourful meals and following functional medicine guidelines is the only preventative option to keeping fit and active well into old age, and the only successful way to treat symptoms of poor health and chronic disease.

After all, we are all made from the food that we eat, so when we fall sick—put simply, there is always a connection somewhere to faulty food, digestion, and poor nutritional balance. Inadequate nutrition can be a major root cause of body systems failing to function correctly.

If we can achieve the same physiological and biochemical effect of drug therapy, by treating chronic disease with nutrients and nutritional supplements (this fact has been extensively researched and medically proven), with no damaging side effects, then why use drugs to treat chronic disease? The obvious answer is profit. Incentives are offered from big pharmaceuticals—and it works.

The myriad biochemical or metabolic pathways within our body systems require dozens of different nutrients daily from a varied diet in order to function efficiently. However, all too often, our body systems are challenged to metabolise processed, unhealthy food and deal with stressful lifestyle habits, resulting in a body that struggles to maintain homeostatic equilibrium—a steady boat, in other words.

Taking a drug for a symptom is like putting a plaster over a sore—ignoring the underlying problem that caused the sore in the first place.

Given the right conditions, the body has a remarkable capacity to heal—it is designed by nature to regenerate itself.

We are all biochemically unique and have different inherited nutritional requirements. And it doesn't end there. Food can have virtually the opposite effect in different individuals. Foods that energise one may cause fatigue in another. As the saying goes, 'One man's food is another man's poison.' This is due not only to our unique and individual metabolism, but the fact that people also metabolise and break down food at different rates, which vary according to specific conditions.

How well we digest and absorb our food depends not only on our genetic makeup, dietary choices, lifestyle factors and stress load, but also other environmental and social factors that determine how our body breaks down food for energy. Each generation can also influence genetic outcomes by changing these factors. For example, if heart disease is rife in your family, you can protect yourself by improving the underlying root causes of this disease.

Drugs do not heal your body—they manage symptoms. Taking action to manage the root causes of your health problems is an area that requires your input. This is the very area where you can take responsibility to improve and maintain your own health. You can contribute to your own healing process and steer the ship—in stark contrast to handing over your body for medication directed by medics who are not generally trained in nutritional medicine.

This is not new-fangled anti-establishment advice, but common sense based on good reputable science that understands the physiology of the human body, and how this works in harmony with the healing power of plant components and nature. It can make the difference between you living in poor health, focusing only on symptom management, or thriving in good health by treating the very causative factors that are linked to disease.

In order to impart usable nutritional knowledge, it has been necessary to go into a little depth in some places on the following pages. However, this book is designed to be an easy-to-follow reference for individuals either with reoccurring minor health problems or those diagnosed with chronic disease. I have included some *cause and effect* examples of how root causes can influence and trigger the development of serious disease. Self-help advice on how to manage distressing symptoms, and help your body to heal naturally, allows you to put in place your own restorative treatment protocols.

By giving you the knowledge to help identify and treat the underlying root causes of your illness, I hope you will be able to regain health and enjoy the freedom and happiness of once again being symptom-free.

Please refer to my other books *Chronic Digestive Disorders* and *On Guard—Boosting Immunity* for a comprehensive understanding of the gut and immune system.

PART I

UNDERSTANDING YOUR BODY

Conventional medicine

The allopathic approach to medical care is to treat the disease, not the person. To treat the symptoms rather than the cause. To compartmentalise the body into specialist areas, which can then be covered in more depth by medical specialists.

The focus is on treating the symptoms of ill health or disease with medication, physiotherapy, or surgery.

For acute medical conditions, emergency medicine and surgical procedures are obviously the only way to save lives and improve immediate health. Drugs save lives. Modern medicine is now so advanced that we can be happy that we do not live in medieval times.

But holistically, the wider picture involving a person's individual biochemistry, genetic makeup, dietary balance, type of lifestyle, and the many other factors that affect health are not generally assessed. This is fully understandable, as these assessments involve time.

However, chronic ill health and disease require a different application. Often taking years to develop, they are always linked to underlying root causes that include a faulty diet, poor digestion, nutritional deficiencies, damaging lifestyle or environmental factors, gut bacterial imbalance, inflammation, or infection. The individuals who suffer from these conditions require a personalised approach to healing, because conventional drug strategies applied to chronic conditions may introduce new symptoms of ill health due to side effects. Furthermore, these strategies fail to address the underlying root causes of disease.

Drug treatment is inappropriate when treating chronic disease, because once an individual has embarked on long-term therapy—and it is mostly long term—the original root causes can be hard to identify. The original plot is lost as biochemistry alters. This is not to say that people on medication have no chance of healing—quite the opposite. If you are one of these individuals, it is even more important to replenish nutrients lost with medication and ensure your body systems are working well. Functional medicine is a perfect option to guide you down this pathway with a view to discontinuing medication if possible.

Unfortunately, the conventional approach to treating chronic disease can also affect your quality of everyday life. Science cannot provide bioidentical and cell-compatible chemical compounds. Drugs are manufactured using synthetic versions of the original active ingredients from plants. These synthetically produced drugs are designed to alter the body's biochemistry to cure the symptoms, but long-term side effects of pharmaceutical drug treatments often mask any signs of original underlying biochemical imbalance. These synthetic compounds challenge the body and can cause negative reactions and damaging side effects when taken long term. They are foreign substances unlike anything found in nature.

There are no two individuals completely alike, both physically and biochemically, even between twins and individual families. As every person has quite unique body chemistry, the 'one pill suits all' method used conventionally to treat chronic disease is not always an ideal approach.

Symptom management with drugs is at the expense of true holistic healing. If the underlying root factors linked to disease are not addressed, how can any healing take place? Drugs cannot initiate a healing process. People are often prescribed pills for life and their life may never be the same afterwards. Paradoxically, it can also lead them on a pathway to further ill health.

Functional medicine

In contrast to conventional medicine, functional medicine, FM for short, treats the person not just the disease—it follows a naturopathic model. It offers the person an individual and personalised healthcare approach that aims to identify the root causes of symptoms at the cellular level, then designing appropriate nutritional protocols to correct imbalance.

Functional medicine treats underlying causes of ill health and focuses on the person holistically. Nature provides us with inbuilt mechanisms to maintain our health and heal the body without the use of synthetic drugs (unless vital use for surgery and emergencies). Treatment strategies are designed to correct nutritional deficiencies, faulty body system function, and imbalanced biochemistry—allowing the innate natural healing processes within the body to respond and heal accordingly.

Functional medicine assesses the function of body systems in depth by laboratory analyses. Practitioners are trained in analysing biochemical tests, which may incorporate standard laboratory medical tests or specialised biochemical and nutritional tests.

Correcting biochemical imbalance with nutrients such as vitamins, amino acids, fatty acids, trace elements and minerals—the very substances the body is composed of—is a truly holistic approach. Plant chemical extracts, medicinal plants and enzyme therapy are amongst other considerations that are used in nutritional medicine.

What can I expect when I visit a functional medicine practitioner?

First and foremost, you will be regarded as an individual. The approach will be personalised, regardless of your presenting symptoms. The symptoms and your medical history are important guidelines for practitioners. The emphasis will be on assessing the function of your body systems and biochemistry linked to your symptoms—using various laboratory tests. Your medical history, presenting symptoms, current and past diet will be analysed together with your lifestyle and living habits, the environment you live and work in, your state of mind and emotions, and your genetic makeup and individual biochemistry—plus every other possible factor that may be linked to your current state of health.

There is no magic bullet offered. The in-depth assessments for the underlying causes of chronic disease, in the form of medical laboratory tests, are not stressful. They provide the practitioner with comprehensive invaluable insights into the internal functioning of your body. Many profiles are user friendly and can be run in the privacy of your own home, such as the Comprehensive Digestive Stool Analysis. If cost is prohibitive, it is possible to achieve many positive changes without the benefit of tests. Some systems may respond well to general advice and recommendations. An experienced practitioner is well aware that any change in the right direction brings immense benefits.

Healing the body holistically means taking action to identify, analyse, unravel, and reverse the steps the body has been through to reach your current state of poor health. It will require your cooperation, time, and dedication to fulfil your side of the healing process. It will be a partnership, a learning process to help you understand how your own body functions and why you are so ill. You will also learn precisely how to make the necessary changes to reverse your current state of poor health.

There will be monthly follow-ups and treatment plans that may be adjusted depending on the progress made. The tests may be repeated post treatment, to ascertain whether improvements have been achieved. Alternatively, if cost is an issue, obvious improvement made and your satisfaction with the process should suffice. Changes should be made slowly and in tune with the metabolic pace of your body as it strives to adjust to a new, healthy you.

You should feel ongoing improvement every step of the way. After the initial process of changing your diet, getting rid of unhealthy habits, and improving any stressful lifestyle, you should enjoy newfound benefits that will give you the inspiration to continue. If, by chance, you feel temporarily unwell, it is a result of the positive changes being made, however odd that sounds. Do not panic and revert back to unhealthy ways. There may be some initial rebound withdrawal effects due to dietary change, especially if you have been addicted to sugar, processed foods, alcohol, and other damaging stimulants over a long period of time. But your body will be learning new ways and it needs time to adapt. A practitioner will guide you through these withdrawal effects if they do appear, as they are vital steps to recovery.

Not everybody has negative reactions. The trick is to work carefully and methodically through the steps that need addressing in tune with your specific metabolic tempo. Recognise this rhythm and don't expect an overnight fix. Having said this, it is also not a good idea to delay the obvious and take weeks to avoid damaging foods or lifestyles. The sooner changes can be made at a happy pace, the quicker your recovery will take place.

Being involved in every step of the process of regaining health can be personally inspiring. You control your own healing process—this can prove a mental tonic and uplifting experience.

Examples of some biochemical laboratory tests used by functional medicine/nutritional therapist practitioners to analyse root causes of ill health:

- Immunology profile
- Nutritional genomics
- Metabolic function
- Organic Acid balance
- Cardiovascular profile
- Amino Acid balance
- Comprehensive Digestive Stool Analysis
- Microbiology Pathogens, parasites, bacteria, and yeast
- Nutritional profile
- Fatty Acids profile
- Inflammatory markers
- GI Effects

- Gut Dysbiosis
- Thyroid profile
- Food Allergy Antibodies
- Health Risk Assessment
- Toxic Heavy Metals
- Elemental Minerals
- Nutritional and Toxic Elements
- Oxidative Stress
- Cognitive Health
- Cardio Metabolic
- Environmental profile
- Autoimmune Reactivity
- Mucosal Immune Reactivity
- Gut-Brain Barrier
- Hormone panel
- Adrenal Stress
- Neurotransmitter profile

As you can see, the list above of biochemical test procedures is quite comprehensive. Obviously, a practitioner would be focusing on the systems linked to your presenting symptoms. The choice of tests to be run lies with the expertise of your practitioner and, as in most of these tests, it is not always a black and white situation. That is the beauty of running comprehensive profiles—they give an overall insight into the state of your body, not just one marker but multiple—all indicating a clearer picture and highlighting areas that may pose a higher risk of disease. They require expert analysis to put all the information together, to recognise the biochemical pathways in each body system, and to build an effective individual treatment plan according to your personal genetic makeup and metabolic function.

What are the root causes of disease?

The root causes of disease can be considered the triggers that send you down a pathway to poor health. Triggers that raise your risk of serious disorders. At the fundamental cellular level, when you become unwell, your body develops changes in your biochemistry and in your physical capacity. The biochemical systems that run your body start to falter and struggle.

Initially, you may not attach much importance to these basic signs of ill health as you head to the chemist or search online for help. It is not always easy to identify triggers, unless you are a professional; but, as the body imbalance continues because the underlying cause has not been dealt with, the risk of poor health spiralling into disease increases.

Chronic ill health is a result of years of suffering—an accumulation of symptoms that overwhelm the body. As with everything in life, prevention and early intervention is better than a cure. Every sign of ill health has a causative factor.

Recognising and investigating the root cause of your health problems at an early stage can help you to recover quickly. But do not despair if your health has been poor for years. You live in a very responsive body, which is designed by nature to keep you fit and well. It runs on healthy fuel (your diet) and, given improved conditions, it will work hard for you to regain your health.

ROOT CAUSES OF DISEASES LINKED TO ILL HEALTH

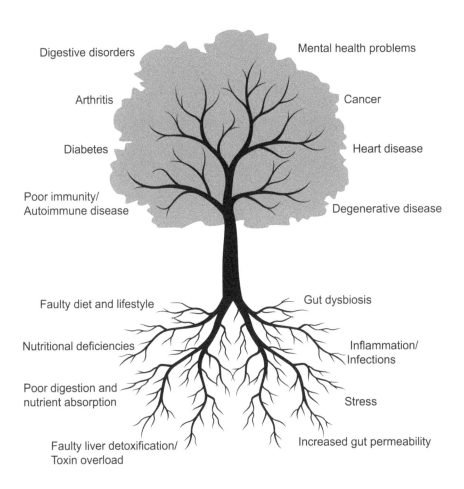

Your body's call for help

Minor symptoms of poor health may not register as warning signs as to what may lay ahead until they become a distinct issue for concern. We rarely feel totally fit day in day out, as our very existence depends not only on internal factors but the external environment around us. We are conditioned to expect low days—off days, recovery days, catch-up sleep after late-night days, or simply days when we feel less energetic as normal.

But there is an accumulative pattern when the body eventually spirals into a permanent state of ill health. And, as there are valid causes for this decline, these issues need addressing before the body can regenerate and heal.

Factors linked to the development of disease:

- Nutrient-deficient food
- Imbalanced diet
- Unhealthy lifestyle
- Toxic overload
- Physical and mental stress
- Poor body repair and renewal of cells
- Dysfunction in body systems
- Disease

After the event, you may look back and link certain accumulative symptoms that have given you cause for worry in the past. You may recognise a cause and effect pattern from your eating habits and lifestyle. With some analytical thought, you may be able to pinpoint a starting point for initiating changes. The basics concerning diet and lifestyle may not initially need the expertise of a practitioner. I would suggest making obvious changes that you feel may be linked to your symptoms; however, if you need further in-depth guidance, seek the advice of a professional. At the latter part of this book are my recommendations for improving diet and lifestyle, for dealing with stress and infection and supporting good digestion.

If you are suffering with a serious diagnosed disease, or have been prescribed medication, then you will require professional help.

Your body cells are being constantly repaired

According to the journal *Scientific American,* it has been estimated that 330 billion cells in our body are replaced daily—practically 1% of the body—and 1 million cells in our body die every second. As published in the original article by Mark Fischetti and Jen Christiansen in April 2021, 'A new you in 80 days.'

All this internal activity requires the correct fuel—the nutrients in your diet. This is why you cannot keep really fit and well without a nutrient-rich diet.

- Your intestinal lining is replaced on average every 3-5 days
- Every 3 months or so, you are effectively a new you, and approximately every 7 years your entire collection of body cells get replaced
- Your hair grows on average 6 inches per year
- Your kidneys filter a litre of blood every minute
- Your immune system cells are renewed weekly
- Your entire red blood cells are replaced every 2-3 months — 2.5 million red blood cells are renewed every second

- Around 40,000 skin cells are replaced every minute
- Your brain cells keep regenerating throughout life, albeit at a slower pace as you age
- Every day, 8 litres of stomach juices are produced to break down your food

As you can see from these figures, you do not remain throughout life with the same body—you are constantly evolving, and you can influence the status quo at any time. *Cell Biology*, Ron Milo, Rob Phillips www.bionumbers.org

Some early signs of poor health

Do you often feel:

- Under the weather?
- Lacking in energy?
- Unrefreshed on waking?
- Stressed and unable to cope with life?
- You have poor hair quality or ridged nails?
- You have unhealthy skin conditions?
- Puffiness under the eyes or have dark rings in the same area?
- Unfit and exhausted after exercise?
- You have difficulty fighting infections?

These are symptoms of poor health that you may never think would be linked to the state of your diet, nutrient balance, and gut health. Other signs may include muscle aches and joint pain, frequent headaches, fatigue, peeling nails, poor eyesight, lanky dry hair or just a general feeling of unwellness.

ACCUMULATIVE FACTORS LEADING TO ILL HEALTH

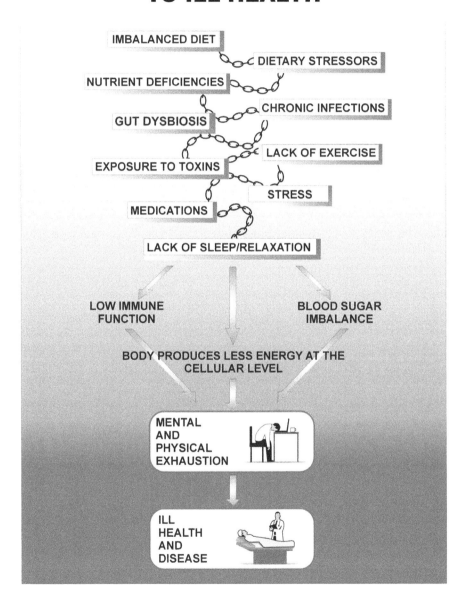

But do not despair—these signs of poor health can often be alleviated and reversed purely by improving your diet, by focusing on organic nutrient-dense foods and optimising the health of your gut.

How you look and feel is the best indicator of the quality of your diet and lifestyle.

Symptoms of ill health do not appear without reason; they are not 'caught' like an infection. They develop over time as a direct result of certain identifiable root causes. You are not sick due to lack of a drug, but due to lack of correct fuel to run your body.

The paradox is that we live in a world full of choice and, in the Western world, an adequate food supply. Yet, because of ignorance about good nutrition and the invasive power of food marketing, many people are unaware of the fact that, by eating processed food, they are in danger of becoming malnourished.

The human body doesn't need the vast mass of food choice available. Degenerative diseases are on the rise and the basic reasons are obvious. There is an epidemic, not of infections, but of chronically sick people. Many exist on medication to keep them reasonably able to cope with life—they are just ticking over—but this does not constitute good health.

Some vitamin and mineral deficiency signs:

VITAMIN A

Mouth ulcers, poor night vision, acne, frequent colds and infections, dry skin, dandruff, diarrhoea, cataracts, and cystitis.

VITAMIN D

Joint pains and stiffness, muscle cramps, backache, tooth decay, hair loss, excessive perspiration, lack of energy, low immunity, and depression.

VITAMIN E

Easy bruising, exhaustion after light exercise, slow wound healing, varicose veins, and a lack of sex drive.

VITAMIN C

Frequent colds and infections, slow wound healing, bleeding and tender gums, easy bruising, and a lack of energy.

VITAMIN B1

Tender muscles, eye pains, irritability, poor concentration and memory loss, prickly legs, tingling hands, stomach pains, and a rapid heartbeat.

VITAMIN B2

Bloodshot/burning/gritty eyes, sensitivity to bright lights, sore tongue, cataracts, dull oily hair, eczema, split nails, and cracked lips.

VITAMIN B3

Lack of energy, insomnia, headaches, anxiety, tension, depression, irritability, and acne.

VITAMIN B5

Muscle tremors, cramps, spasms in legs, apathy, poor concentration, stress, burning feet, tender heels, and nausea.

Gaynor J Greber

SYMPTOMS OF MAGNESIUM DEFICIENCY

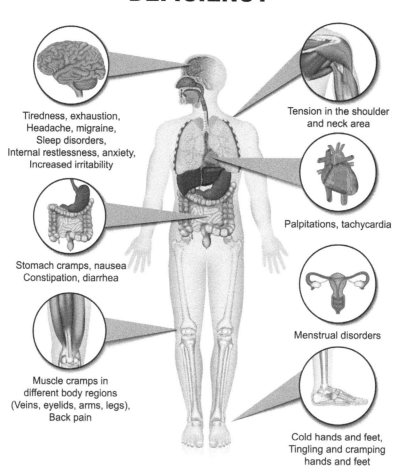

Tiredness, exhaustion,
Headache, migraine,
Sleep disorders,
Internal restlessness, anxiety,
Increased irritability

Stomach cramps, nausea
Constipation, diarrhea

Muscle cramps in
different body regions
(Veins, eyelids, arms, legs),
Back pain

Tension in the shoulder
and neck area

Palpitations, tachycardia

Menstrual disorders

Cold hands and feet,
Tingling and cramping
hands and feet

VITAMIN B6

Infrequent dream recall, PMT, water retention, tingling hands, panic attacks, depression, irritability, nervous disorders, digestive complaints, and a lack of energy.

VITAMIN B12

Pale skin, constipation, sensitive tongue, poor hair condition, anaemia, nerve dysfunction/tingling, numbness in extremities, sore arms and legs, and psychological and neurological problems.

FOLIC ACID

Low appetite, cracked lips, depression, poor memory, and low energy.

CALCIUM and MAGNESIUM

Muscle cramps, palpitations, insomnia, stress, tooth decay, high blood pressure, and the inability to relax.

ZINC

Loss of taste and smell, stretch marks, white marks on nails, frequent infections, digestive problems, hormonal dysfunction, acne and skin conditions, panic attacks, anxiety, and stress.

IRON

Pale skin, sore tongue, loss of appetite, nausea, ridges on nails, spoon-shaped nails, and anaemia.

COPPER

Hair loss and loss of hair colour and skin pigmentation, heart disorders, and panic attacks.

SYMPTOMS OF SELENIUM DEFICIENCY

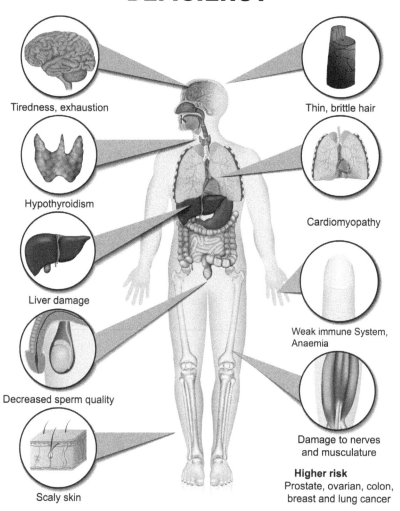

Tiredness, exhaustion

Hypothyroidism

Liver damage

Decreased sperm quality

Scaly skin

Thin, brittle hair

Cardiomyopathy

Weak immune System, Anaemia

Damage to nerves and musculature

Higher risk
Prostate, ovarian, colon, breast and lung cancer

CHROMIUM

Blood sugar imbalance, sugar cravings, lack of energy, and stress.

POTASSIUM

Irregular heartbeat, muscle spasms and twitches, insomnia, fluid retention, menstrual problems, anxiety, and thyroid problems.

ESSENTIAL FATTY ACIDS—OMEGA 3-6-9

Dry skin, skin disorders, poor eyesight, hormonal imbalance, nervous conditions, and mental instability.

Naturally, there are many other factors that can cause similar symptoms. But when deficiencies exist, your body is obviously being short-changed within your diet. Nutrition keeps us alive and in a state of wellness. You wouldn't think of short-changing your car with the wrong type of fuel.

We require a vast array of nutrients on a daily basis, so it is not advisable to supplement odd nutrients that you may have read about, hoping to gain some health benefit. You need at least a quality multi-vitamin and mineral product as a basic product if you are taking supplements, coupled with a varied diet to supply these nutrients. It is all about balance and harmony. All nutrients work synergistically together in the body. This means they each have various co-factor minerals and vitamins that enhance absorption and aid biochemical function.

For example, zinc and vitamin B6 are required for the production of stomach acid and insulin, for regulating mood and sleep patterns, for healthy brain function and energy metabolism. Chromium and vitamin B3, calcium and magnesium, copper and zinc, and selenium and vitamin E are other examples of nutrients that work together in various metabolic processes. Another example is vitamin C. If we consider its vital role in skin repair and wound healing, it works together with zinc and also has an improved effect when bioflavonoids are added to the formula.

Many health problems can be caused or exacerbated by mineral imbalance:

- Chromium, manganese, and magnesium deficiency can lead to diabetes
- Zinc deficiency can lead to mental health problems
- High levels of copper can lead to schizophrenia or hormonal disturbance
- Magnesium deficiency can lead to heart disease and musculo-skeletal problems

Some damaging effects of heavy metal toxicity

Heavy metal toxicity can occur from environmental or workplace contamination, surgical metal implants, dental appliances and fillings, vaccines, aluminium cans, and cooking utensils.

Heavy metals displace minerals in cellular binding sites and contribute to the following health disorders:

- Copper—mental health or hormonal problems
- Lead and Mercury—arthritis, neuro-degenerative disease, hyperactivity, mental health problems
- Cobalt—cancer, heart disease, hypertension, stroke

- Aluminium—dementia, kidney or liver damage, muscle weakness, seizures

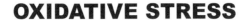

OXIDATIVE STRESS

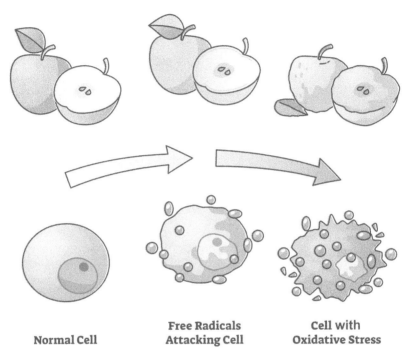

Normal Cell	**Free Radicals Attacking Cell**	**Cell with Oxidative Stress**

What are free radicals and antioxidants?

Free radicals are reactive molecules that attack cells, DNA, and the fatty acid structure of cell walls. Free radical damage has been linked to accelerated aging, degenerative diseases, heart disease, arthritis, cancer, and autoimmune disorders.

This damage can occur when you eat burnt or barbecued food, eat hydrogenated or partially hydrogenated oils that have had their molecular structure altered by processing, or when you are exposed to toxins in food or in the environment. Intensive physical training can also stress the body, exposing an individual to free radical damage and making them more liable to pick up infections. This can lead to poor immunity.

The good news is that our bodies are well equipped to scavenge and disarm these free radicals. We have enzyme systems that inhibit the formation of damaging molecules and keep cells healthy. These enzyme systems are dependent on nutrients and antioxidants found in our food supply. Antioxidants are nutrients that deactivate free radicals and protect the body from any destructive activity in the cell membranes.

There are hundreds of antioxidants found in food and plants. Some are nutrients, for example vitamins A, C, and E, zinc, selenium, co-enzyme Q10, alpha lipoic acid and beta carotene. Others found in plants include bioflavonoids, anthocyanidins, lycopene, lutein and other pigments and non-essential plant chemicals that have a role in supporting the body's immune system.

Eating colourful fresh foods rich in antioxidants is always the best support you can give your immune system—collectively, these are called phytochemicals.

Eating a varied colourful rainbow diet rich in onions, garlic, nuts, seeds, whole grains, beans, and fruit (especially black and red berries and green vegetables), including foods containing the amino acids (protein) glutathione and cysteine that function as antioxidants (found in fish, light meat and dairy products), can help keep your body in optimum health.

Why should I eat organic?

The produce from fields, unless organically grown, is drenched with chemical pesticides and herbicides throughout the growing seasons, with often repeated spraying to produce a higher yield.

These toxic chemicals have hormone-altering effects on human cells and can accumulate in the soil. Post-harvest, there may be cosmetic spraying to polish up the fruit and make it more desirable when on display in the marketplace.

One study back in 1995 showed that 18% of lettuces and 30% of milk products contained pesticide residues, and 82% of UK-produced chocolate contained residues of a dangerous chemical called lindane (related to DDT). This is banned in 14 countries and linked to breast cancer. *Food Magazine Oct-Dec 1995.*

Despite this being an old study, pesticide residues are still being found in food produce grown today by conventional intensive farming practices.

Currently, due to the goalposts having been moved, there are legally approved raised limits for pesticide residues! Residues are still evident, but mostly within the new set limits based on an arbitrary whim and a need for profit. There should be no limits set by man for toxins entering our food chain.

Eating organic is the only healthy way forward.

The increase in organic farming practices is encouraging. Organic produce is more nutritious, has more flavour and is dense in nutrients.

https://bio-nichtbio.info is a German site that produces images of the life force found in fruit and vegetables. Photographed with special Kilian photography, the difference between organic and conventional images is stark. The wonderful book *Bio and Nichtbio* tells it all in vivid, stunning, full-page pictures—it is a treasure to have and a reminder to eat organic.

Organic produce is healthier for your body, especially for the sick who require the highest quality calories.

The benefits of eating organic:

Produce is higher in nutrients than in conventionally grown produce.

The nutrients are denser and richer with antioxidants that have anti-aging effects and help protect against cancer and degenerative diseases.

Hens fed on organic food produce richer more nutritious eggs.

The crops taste better as flavour comes from nutrients extracted from healthy soil, and the structure of organic plants is stronger as a result.

The produce keeps fresh longer at room temperature as the active enzymes are intact and the produce contains less water.

Crops grown in fertile, replenished soil enhance ecological balance of the natural world.

The rotation of crops helps prevent plant disease and builds up soil fertility.

Eating organic reduces your exposure to damaging chemicals used in intensive conventional farming: heavy metals, pesticides, herbicides, artificial fertilisers, organophosphates. These include antibiotics, synthetic hormones, and drugs used in dairy farming and sewage sludge used as fertiliser on agricultural land.

According to various articles from the water industry in the UK, 78% of treated human faeces and solid sludge is spread over the land yearly. Medications and synthetic hormones pass through bodies and can land up in waterways or on the land.

PART II

UNDERSTANDING THE ROOT CAUSES OF DISEASE AND CAUSE AND EFFECT CONSIDERATIONS

THE GUT

Your intestinal tract—the gut—is the cornerstone of good health.

If your gut is unhealthy, this will certainly have a knock-on effect on all of your body systems.

Poor digestion and absorption of nutrients can raise the risk of bowel cancer and other serious diseases.

Maldigestion

If you are not breaking down your food efficiently, this condition is called maldigestion.

Many people may consider rumbles, gurgles, and flatulence in the gut to be the norm, or that being constipated is just one of those inconveniences that will eventually get better. These symptoms, however minor, are telling you that all is not well. Producing fermenting gas in the gut indicates you are not breaking down and digesting your food properly or are reacting to unhealthy, processed food such as sugar. Constipation generally indicates dehydration, low levels of dietary fibre in your diet, lack of exercise, magnesium, or vitamin C deficiency.

SYMPTOMS OF DYSBIOSIS

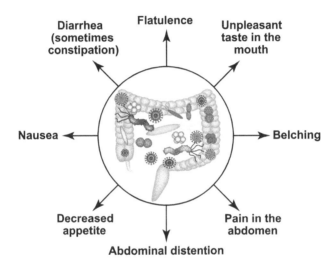

It has been estimated that every third person in the Western world has had some type of chronic digestive complaint in the past few months and many people suffer with chronic digestive problems life-long. This sounds like really bad news, but the good news is that reversing the stages the body went through to develop an unhealthy gut can also miraculously restore and heal the intestinal tract.

How healthy is your digestive system?

Do you suffer with the following health problems?

- Irritable bowel syndrome (IBS)

- Indigestion, bad breath, or burping after meals
- Flatulence, bloating, or stomach cramps after eating
- Constipation, diarrhoea, or greasy foul-smelling stools
- Frequent bouts of heartburn or discomfort after eating
- Chronic fatigue or skin conditions

WHY GUT HEALTH MATTERS

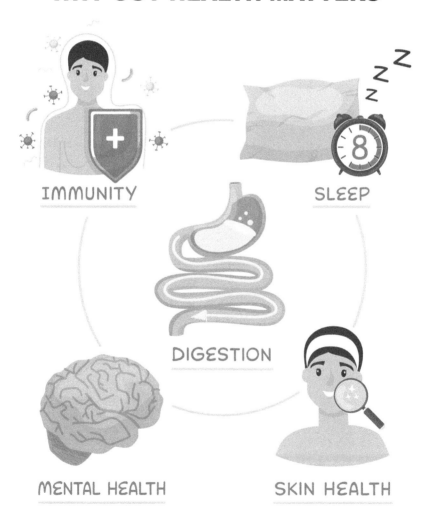

Digestive complaints can range from minor but distressing symptoms such as bloating, flatulence, indigestion, heartburn, and food intolerances to serious disorders including Coeliac disease, ulcers, gastritis, colitis, ulcerative colitis, irritable bowel syndrome and Crohn's disease.

Faulty digestion can have a profound effect on your health. As already explained—your gut feeds every system in your body. It is always the first area that needs addressing if you are looking to analyse the root causes of your health problems.

The body always strives for equilibrium in order for your metabolism to work well. You will be giving your body the biggest gift by correcting unhealthy dietary practices.

Your digestive system rules the entire body. If this system is not functioning properly, all your organs will not be getting the nutrients they require in order to function well. This situation can certainly lead, in time, to poor health. To understand the importance of a healthy gut, ask yourself whether you generally feel comfortable after meals, only occasionally having an upset stomach when you eat the wrong food, or do you live with a chronic range of digestive complaints that never seem to clear up, regardless of any dietary changes you make to improve matters? Self-help can sometimes worsen the situation. You may consider you have a food intolerance and need to avoid certain important necessary food groups. Eating a limited variety of food does not necessarily lead to improved health.

Delayed reactions to food can occur up to three days after you have eaten the suspect item, so you may have little success chasing the culprit. The build-up to maldigestion is an accumulative matter. It can start with a twinge and, on getting ignored and fed further by damaging food, move quickly on to a strong cramp. The more factors involved, the more difficult it will be for you to decipher the starting point.

The best way forward is to see a competent functional medicine practitioner or nutritional therapist who can evaluate your diet and digestive function by running some antibody tests. Assessing true allergies as opposed to food intolerance will allow you to introduce missing healthy foods back into your diet, thus improving your whole eating experience.

If you are able to identify a cause and effect reaction to unhealthy food or drink, you need to make a determined effort to avoid these substances and seek professional advice. Take heed of triggers and pointers. I have been consulted on a few occasions by individuals who, having regained good health, were determined to repeat bad habits and start the whole procedure over again by reintroducing harmful foods and returning to damaging lifestyles. They did not have the willpower to withstand peer pressure, or maybe felt a need to prove a point of view that the body can be controlled by thought processes. They never won; the old symptoms returned with a vengeance and back they were again in my clinic.

When you think about it, it is highly impressive that the human body can heal itself and alerts us when all is not well. It gives warning signs whilst tolerating dietary abuse, but continues to limp along on substandard food, trying to keep your body healthy until, miraculously, it springs back into action as soon as it receives the right response from you.

Naturally, peer pressure plays a big part in young people's lives. Human nature is such that the pleasure of unhealthy treats far outweighs suffering any negative effects. Perhaps enjoying some aspects of the benefits of improved health, such as shiny hair, strong nails, or beautiful skin, can convince others in a group that living healthily does not involve being a killjoy, but is worthwhile, motivating, and inspiring.

Roll back decades and look at the diseases suffered by man — many a direct result of the type of diet eaten. In the Edwardian and Victorian ages, the diet was rich, high in protein and low in fresh vegetables and fruit. There were enormous meals with many rich courses. Gout in those days — a disease linked with high uric acid from purine-rich animal protein foods — was rampant. It still is a diet-related condition, but is now hardly evident at the scale of those days. Kidney stones, gallstones, liver disorders and heart disease were also common for those on rich diets and continue to be a risk for individuals eating a high animal protein acidic diet.

How food gets digested

Every meal you eat prompts the body to produce stomach acid and digestive enzymes to digest the food and prepare it for absorption. We cannot use food in the form that is eaten. Food in its original state needs to be broken down into the smallest possible molecules for the body to absorb and use in cells for energy production, cell repair and maintenance. Hence the need to chew well and start this process as soon as the food is eaten.

The nutrients released by these digestive processes get absorbed mostly in the small intestine. Hydrochloric acid, the stomach acid, helps digest protein in the early stages of the digestive process. The acid environment then stimulates the production of alkaline juices by the pancreas further down the intestinal tract. These juices contain digestive enzymes to finish the task of digesting the meal. Digestion takes place in many stages until all food is adequately broken down into a simple state that allows absorption. But even at this stage, nutrients are vital as co-factors to aid absorption into cells.

Digestive enzymes:

Amylase digests carbohydrates and starches.

A deficiency results in poor energy production in cells.

Protease digests protein.

A deficiency results in an inability to repair and maintain cell walls.

Lipase digests fats.

A deficiency results in poor cell renewal and maintenance.

Consider also that the human body's enzyme system is designed to recognise healthy wholefoods grown by nature. Not gene-altered or processed food. When confronted by man-made concoctions often laden with artificial chemicals, digestion may be incomplete, leaving undigested matter to ferment in the gut.

Factors that influence stomach acid and digestive enzyme production

There are many causes that can interfere with digestive function—aging, nutrient deficiencies, exposure to dietary and environmental toxins, processed food, and high-temperature cooking practices. Enzymes work best within a particular temperature range.

Stress—prolonged and sustained stress, in particular—puts a huge burden on digestive processes as digestion switches off during stress, thereby allowing the central nervous system to deal with the situation. Over time, this can reduce stomach acid output and interfere with enzyme production. Mineral balance can also be affected by acidic changes in cells that occur when a stress-related adrenalin rush stimulates acidic conditions in cells.

Zinc and vitamin B6, required for stomach acid production, are the very nutrients that are depleted when you are under stress. Many individuals lack sufficient nutrient levels, due to the stress cycle depleting B vitamins, magnesium, manganese, zinc, and vitamin C—nutrients required to break down food efficiently. It becomes a vicious cycle—nutrient deficiency causes stress and stress causes nutrient deficiencies. Vitamin C, magnesium, and the B vitamin complex support healthy adrenal function. Those on long-term medication may be at a disadvantage as drug metabolism affects nutrient balance.

Beneficial bugs in your gut

Good absorption of nutrients also requires a healthy balance of beneficial bacteria in the gut.

The gut microbiota, which should consist of mostly healthy bacteria, is a collection of many types of microorganisms including viruses, yeasts, and bacteria—both healthy and unhealthy varieties. When in a healthy state, this microbiota keeps our body in good health. The friendly bacteria help liver detoxification, fight infections, synthesise some vitamins in the gut, and help us absorb minerals. About 25% of our immune system cells also reside in the gut lining; therefore, keeping your gut in top form will help support healthy immune function.

Healthy bacteria coat the intestinal lining. They live in a mucus matrix that protects the sensitive gut lining from infection and damage by dietary toxins and unhealthy microbes. This microbial colony contains friendly lactobacillus species in the small bowel and friendly bifidobacteria species in the large bowel.

Stressors can disturb this army of beneficial bacteria

Many factors can have a negative effect on your intestinal microbial balance—ranging from unresolved stress, alcohol dependency, sugar addiction, poor diet, infections, and illness, as well as the overuse of antibiotics, prescribed medication, stimulants, and toxins.

It is futile searching for the cause, as it can be complex. However, identifying biochemic imbalance with functional medicine tests can give you a precise picture of the status in your gut and the type of support required.

Life in the fast lane –The sugar roller coaster

There is often confusion about sugar. All carbohydrates contain both simple and complex sugars—grains, fruit, vegetables, and starchy foods all metabolise down after digestion into the various natural sugars that the body needs for energy production.

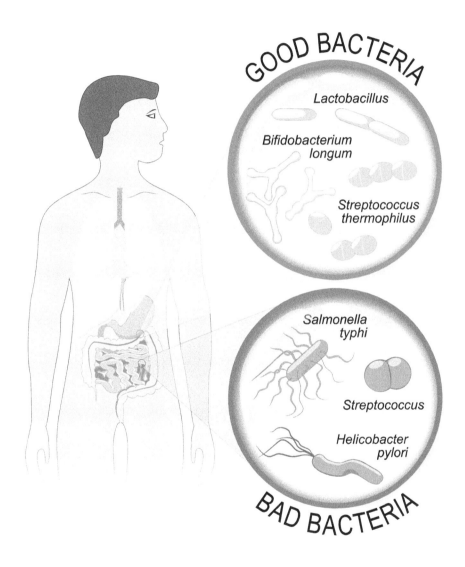

Sugar effects

It is cane sugar that has the most damaging effect on body systems. Bacteria, both friendly and non-friendly species, thrive on sugar. This hits the bloodstream rapidly, disrupting the gut microflora, promoting an overgrowth of unhealthy bacteria, and creating havoc in every body system.

Cane sugar, in any form, is high in calories, addictive, lacks nutritive value and is a major stressor on your hormonal system. Studies have shown that as little as a few teaspoons of sugar can deplete the efficacy of your white blood cells for many hours. This irreplaceable white army is your defence against infection, so sugar puts you at increased risk of infections.

Sugar gives a quick energy fix, but the body retaliates and pays you back a few hours later by dropping your blood sugar levels drastically, prompting sugar cravings. Physical and mental stress rises when the batteries run low and addictive sugar cravings become the norm. A seesaw effect of fluctuating blood sugar levels stresses both body and mind.

Insulin, the glucose hormone, directs cells to absorb glucose for energy making. This hormone is on overdrive in individuals addicted to sugar. Finally, the body may become exhausted and stop reacting to insulin—then diabetes sets in. Prior to type 2 diabetes (dietary related) development, glucose intolerance and insulin resistance (otherwise called syndrome X) can take you down the same pathway. In these conditions, the body starts to turn excess carbohydrates (sugars) that are not absorbed—into fat. This then poses a major health risk for heart disease, as fat is deposited around the heart and in the blood vessels.

INSULIN RESISTANCE

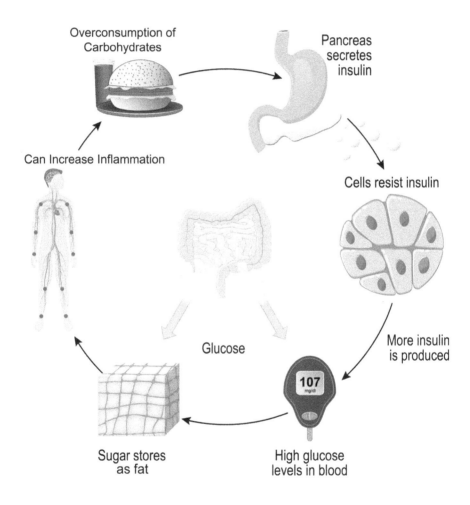

Excess sugar increases weight by being deposited in brown fat cells, particularly around the abdomen. It requires a huge amount of willpower to reduce harmful carbohydrate consumption such as sugar and alcohol, the latter of which is fermented sugar, which disrupts gut bacteria causing dysbiosis. Often, a heart attack is the first shock that brings change to mind.

Your zinc and vitamin B6 stores are used up for insulin production every time you eat sugar. PMS and other hormonal health problems can occur when these nutrient levels drop, as zinc and vitamin B6 are also required for the sex hormones. The more sugar eaten—the more hormonal mayhem.

Sugar, as also mentioned, feeds bacteria and can increase the risk of fungal, viral, or bacterial overgrowth. If dietary or microbial toxins enter the bloodstream, they can activate an immune response and result in autoimmune disease where the body attacks its own cells—rheumatoid arthritis, lupus, multiple sclerosis, type 1 diabetes, Hashimoto's, and Graves' disease, to name a few. More and more studies show a distinct relationship between chronic disease and health of the gut.

Other damaging stressors

Dark strong tea, regular alcohol intake, chocolate, and strong coffee can have the same effect as sugar as far as hormones are concerned. The highs and lows of blood sugar balance—a seesaw effect—can happen with any stimulant. The occasional indulgence is not a big issue. This is tolerated by the body's inbuilt protective mechanisms. But if you regularly eat and drink stimulatory foods or have bad habits, you can expect strong gut reactions.

GUT HEALTH AND BRAIN CONNECTION

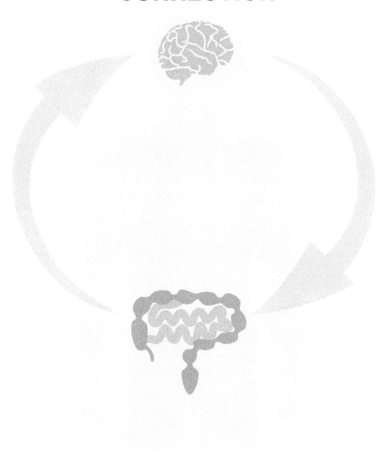

Cigarettes are highly addictive and contain thousands of toxic substances. The liver has to detoxify these dangerous chemicals and, in doing so, uses up reserves of vital nutrients stored in the body.

You eat to maintain and sustain health. But if your diet is imbalanced and you fail to digest your food properly, cells will not be nourished, and repair cannot take place.

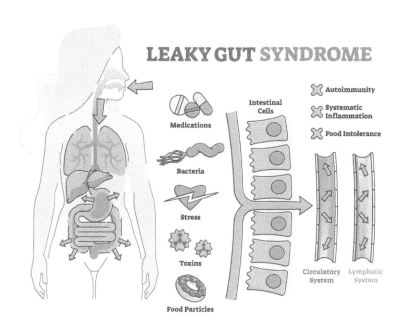

Health consequences of impaired digestion:

- Inflammatory Bowel Disease
- Toxic bowel
- Chronic nutrient deficiencies
- Imbalanced gut bacteria
- Autoimmune Disease
- Allergies and food intolerance

- Leaky gut syndrome (increased gut permeability)
- Immune dysfunction
- Infection

The gut is linked to the brain by biochemical signalling pathways. Mental health, therefore, depends on the state of your gut microbiota. Toxins from the gut can also travel to the brain and cause neurological conditions.

The brain requires adequate zinc, magnesium and vitamins A, B, C, D and K to keep healthy, and manganese, chromium, and vitamin B3 together with other nutrients to balance blood sugar levels that keep the brain happy.

Nausea and headaches can occur when stagnant material is withheld in the gut. As more meals follow, the situation can become chronic with the development of a toxic bowel. There may not be a disease evident, but there is certainly malfunction that needs addressing.

Absence of disease does not mean you are functioning well.

How nutritional deficiencies, excesses, and pH balance influence health.

The pH balance is the acid/alkaline balance in your blood, which is determined by the type of food you eat, which then influences the state of your nervous system.

After metabolism, all foods leave a residual ash that is either alkaline or acidic. The human body cells are naturally slightly alkaline, so if you eat an overly acid-forming diet that is rich in protein, dairy, red meat, alcohol, sugar, tea and coffee, your body's natural status alters. Acidic conditions can lead to inflammation and pain. When the blood becomes too acidic, the body loses the alkaline minerals—calcium, magnesium, potassium, and sodium. These are used to mop up the acidity. Stress also contributes to acid production.

This is one cause of osteoporosis—a typical example of a root cause of disease, where acidic conditions cause the body to draw calcium and magnesium out of the skeletal system to de-acidify the blood.

An unhealthy gut can be linked to skin complaints

Nutritious dietary choices, good digestion and absorption, and healthy gut bacteria are the main criteria for healthy skin.

Skin renewal can only take place with sufficient zinc and vitamin C in the diet. B vitamins are also vitally involved in this process. Years ago, scurvy was found to be caused by a lack of vitamin C in the diet, and beriberi or pellagra skin diseases were caused by a lack of essential fatty acids and B vitamins. When this was discovered, sailors were given citrus fruit to correct this deficiency, and white polished rice was replaced with wholegrain rice, which contained the full range of B vitamins.

Your skin matters, so taking good care of it is very important. It is the largest organ in the human body with many vital functions:

- As a protective waterproof barrier for all internal organs
- As an insulator to regulate body temperature and loss of moisture
- As a private climate control for your internal environment
- As a manufacturer of vitamin D from sunshine
- As a sensory organ to indicate pain

- As an organ of excretion together with the lungs, kidneys, and bowel

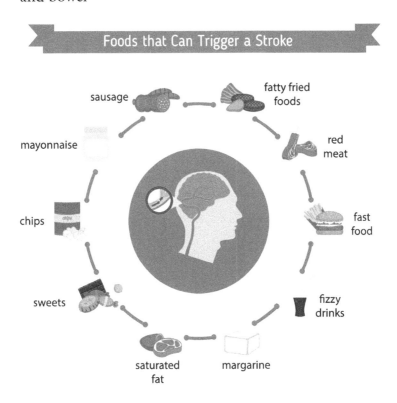

The skin is subject to many changes throughout life, such as during puberty, pregnancy and in advanced age. Bumps, blisters, and rashes appear and disappear, mostly depending on your general state of health. Your skin indicates the health of your inner organs. Food intolerances, allergies, infections, and reactions to mould, chemicals, cosmetics, drugs, and alcohol can all leave their mark. Free radical damage causes skin wrinkling, but there are compounds in certain plants –pigments called proanthocyanins, as well as the polyphenol compounds in grape seed and pine bark—that can help reduce free radical damage. Eating sulphur-rich foods and supplementing with these pigments can help prevent further tissue damage and improve your skin's appearance.

The condition of the skin can suggest many internal health problems. Most aspects of faulty living affect the skin. It can lead to premature aging and practitioners can get a general idea of an individual's health by studying their skin. Puffiness and a discolouration under the eyes can often indicate liver and gallbladder problems, as well as poor digestive or detoxification function. Signs of fatigue and stress and poor adrenal function can be seen in dark circles under the eyes.

Nutritional deficiencies can be linked to poor eye health

Macular degeneration, dry eye syndrome, cataracts, conjunctivitis, retinitis pigmentosa and other eye conditions respond well to nutritional treatment.

Eyes keep healthy with the right nutrients. If these nutrients are lacking in your diet or are not digested and absorbed well, eye disorders can develop.

Inflammation in the gut can be linked to heart disease

Inflammatory processes start in the gut. Refer to my book *Chronic Digestive Disorders.*

Coronary heart disease is the leading cause of death in the Western world. The sad thing is that heart disease is preventable. Research has linked heart disease with inflammation.

Your heart is the most important muscle in your body. It needs regular exercise to keep it in perfect condition and a healthy diet to supply heart protective nutrients.

Hypertension, clogged arteries, arrhythmias, and heart failure are all avoidable diseases.

Nutritional medicine can deal with all of the root causes of cardiovascular heart disease, but it is far better to avoid them in the first place and live a moderate, healthy lifestyle.

One example of the support nutritional medicine can give is the use of minerals to treat palpitations and arrhythmias. When magnesium supplementation is taken to relax the heart muscle, palpitations settle down. The heart muscle fibrillates due to a faulty calcium/magnesium balance in the heart muscle—this causes an imbalance in the nervous system cells, the messaging that takes place between nerve endings.

Calcium contracts the heart muscle and magnesium relaxes it. If there is imbalance between these two minerals, coupled with an imbalance between potassium and sodium that operates the little pump system in cells called the sodium potassium pump, then the muscle can fibrillate. These minerals are called electrolytes and they control the electrical activity of your body—this is very important for the heart muscle. Magnesium also controls the sodium/potassium pump, so this mineral has a leading role to play.

It is common for individuals to be deficient in magnesium—it is used up in the stress cycle together with zinc and B vitamins. Suffering with palpitations and arrhythmias is an indication that the nervous system is under stress.

On occasion, palpitations can be the result of having a large, fatty meal as the stomach lies close to the heart. This can mimic signs of heart distress. Undigested food or fermented gas may also be the culprit.

Atherosclerosis and arteriosclerosis are diseases directly linked to poor dietary balance and use of dietary stimulants. Even if you have a family history of such disorders, your body can avoid developing the same diseases if you take action to eat in a healthy fashion and avoid the commonly recognised factors that can lead to heart disease. Genetics play a small part of this risk, but it is the expression of your genes that is determined by your diet and lifestyle that increases this risk.

Many cases of cardiovascular disease are in an advanced state by the time they present to medics. However, even then, there are many healing procedures to follow to prevent further damage.

There are various types of intravenous 'chelation' therapies that attempt to hoover out the plaque that narrows the arteries, but prevention is always better than cure because there are risks attached to these procedures. Fragments of plaque can potentially block the blood flow and cause more damage.

Enzyme therapy is an alternative treatment to help clear plaque. Used together with other guidelines mentioned—plus a monitored exercise programme—it can work wonders to clear arteries and reverse cardiovascular disease.

Dietary changes can definitely help to reabsorb plaque and stop further build-up. Even just increasing your water intake and exercising can start the process back to recovery.

It is not just diet that predisposes an individual to heart disease. Other factors such as stress, lifestyle and genetic makeup, the acid/alkaline balance in tissues, body types such as fast or slow metabolisers, nutritional status, body inflammation, blood sugar imbalance, and the level of oxidised fats in the body all play a part.

Nutritional deficiencies, toxins, infection and digestive disorders can be linked to infertility and miscarriage

Do you suffer from bacterial overgrowth, allergies, food intolerance, digestive or bowel conditions, or general poor health?

Fungal overgrowth or bacterial/viral infections in the gut can affect fertility and the ability to carry a foetus to full term.

Over 80% of the population have been found to be deficient in certain nutrients. This is not surprising, since modern diets often lack healthy levels of these vital elements.

Nutrients play a vital role in fertility. All nutrients are important, but the key players are the B vitamins, vitamins C and A, and zinc. The amino acids from protein are also necessary for the production of sex hormones.

Investigating the root causes of infertility means stripping back to fundamentals:

- Choice and quality of diet
- Digestion and absorption
- Effects of environmental toxins (anti-nutrients)
- Damaging lifestyle — alcohol, smoking, drugs (anti-nutrients)
- Medication
- Hormonal imbalance due to nutrient deficiency

Nutritional deficiencies can contribute to:

- **Low sperm count and motility**
- **Miscarriage, stillbirth, premature birth, and foetal deformities**

During many years' practice as a Foresight Practitioner for Infertility and Preconceptual care, I witnessed numerous success stories. Many were babies born from healthy parents who had followed my recommended programmes.

THE LIVER

Your liver is the largest organ in your body and has a major role in ensuring that any incoming nutrients reach the cells and toxic waste is eliminated. If its function is compromised, this can lead to general poor health and serious disease patterns. Liver dysfunction can, therefore, be a major root cause of disease as it plays a major part in keeping us healthy.

The human body has inbuilt detoxification pathways, and the liver is in charge of this task, but it does have limits. Modern diets containing processed and refined foods laden with artificial additives, preservatives, flavour enhancers and other foreign chemicals that can damage our cells stress the liver. Nature provides us with mechanisms to metabolise toxins and get rid of the waste, but the higher the load, the more stress the liver undergoes.

It is the storage site for certain vitamins and minerals—iron and copper, vitamins A, B12, D, E, and K—providing them to cells when needed, or to be used when the body stores run low.

Liver function:

- Helps with the formation of red blood cells
- Performs tasks that break down food for energy and converts nutrients into usable forms for absorption

- Converts toxic waste into less dangerous forms, ready to pass down the elimination pathways

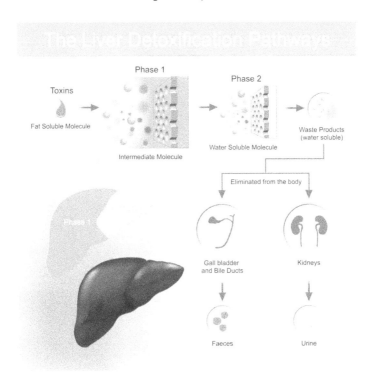

Your liver is a wonder organ. It can miraculously regenerate itself—even after 90% of it has been removed.

One of the most important functions it controls is detoxification. The human body is challenged every day by harmful substances. We are exposed to thousands of foreign chemicals in the environment and in our food supply.

How wonderful it is that nature has provided us with the means to clear out these harmful non-food substances from our body.

The liver converts these into less harmful compounds and shunts them off for excretion. There are two phases of operation in the liver. These phases are run by enzymes, which are dependent on nutrients—mainly amino acids. The phases are called the P-450 system. It converts and excretes toxins, drugs, alcohol, and any other substance that is harmful to the body.

Individual amino acids have many other functions apart from facilitating liver detoxification:

- Improving wound healing
- Improving muscle and joint repair
- Increasing sperm count
- Enhancing fat burning
- Balancing blood fats
- Controlling weight and appetite satiety
- Improving hair/skin and nail growth
- Scavenging free radicals and protecting organs and cells from damage
- Improving mental alertness and memory loss
- Restoring a damaged gut lining
- Reducing fat accumulation in the liver and supporting bile production
- Acting as antioxidants, antidepressants, and pain relievers
- Detoxifying excess histamine and oestrogen
- Increasing the release of growth hormone
- Supporting a healthy heart, helping heart muscle contraction and blood pressure balance
- Offering protection from eye disorders

Toxic overload can hinder your body's use of nutrients gained from a healthy diet.

Toxic elements such as heavy metals—aluminium, mercury, lead, cobalt, and chromium—displace minerals by occupying the mineral-binding sites in cells.

These heavy metals can be in our water supply, in our mouths as dental implants, bridges, etc, or in our surgically implanted metal joint replacements. Ceramic prosthetics are always bio compatible and much healthier.

Always check with your doctor and dentist that the materials they use are not over time poisoning you!

There are biological dentists available in many countries, and doctors who care enough to choose products for surgery that help mitigate any negative effects that their patients may experience in the future.

In the USA, over 80,000 toxic chemicals are found in the food supply, and in Europe the situation is not much better. In 2020, researchers at Brunel University in London in the UK found over 12,000 hazardous carcinogenic and mutagenic materials listed on food packaging alone.

Toxins to avoid:

Metals used in dentistry. Mercury, one of the deadliest most toxic elements on earth, has been permanently fixed into our mouths for decades and is still being used by the NHS in the UK.

Mercury and aluminium. These toxic metals have been used in vaccinations formulas, particularly for babies and children.

Produce saturated with herbicides and pesticides. Rivers are polluted with toxic waste. These chemicals function as hormone disruptors.

Gases, industrial vapours, and toxic fumes.

Drinking water polluted by industry.

Damaging chemicals in cleaning products and personal body care items.

Worldwide vaccine use exposes individuals to a cocktail of additives. Individuals can react not only to the active virus or bacterial material but also to the adjuvants added to stop a serious reaction—aluminium, sugars, gelatine, formaldehyde, antibiotics, preservatives, mercury, squalene, foetal calf serum, human foetal serum and other animal tissue, emulsifiers, MSG flavour enhancer and polysorbates. All these products have been used in various vaccine formulas. Is it any wonder that the side effects from vaccines are played down in the name of profit by multi-pharmaceutical giants?

The human body should not be continuously under physical chronic stress due to the toxins that are absorbed on a daily basis.

It doesn't stop there. New vaccines are being touted every year for every known disease. We do have a very efficient immune system (not profit-making, of course), but this is pushed aside. The powers that be maintain that, without vaccines, we cannot protect ourselves!

The only way of naturally boosting immunity is with the supplementary use of nutrients, medicinal plants, and a super-charged diet full of the antioxidants and phytochemicals found in colourful fruit and vegetables. Nature provides everything we need for immune support.

Faulty liver function can be linked to neurological and mental disorders

There are a range of diseases including multiple sclerosis, Parkinson's disease, Alzheimer's disease, dementia, and ALS (Amyotrophic Lateral Sclerosis) that are linked to multiple causative effects, including poor liver function.

Throughout life, one may have been exposed to toxic heavy metals, often from dental materials or vaccinations. An individual may have had environmental exposure to chemicals containing pesticides and herbicides, perhaps even in their own garden. Generally, these serious diseases could be a result of profound exposure, coupled with other factors. Consider mercury. How much of this deadly poison was put in people's mouths all in the name of repairing teeth?

Why were babies and children injected with vaccines containing mercury and aluminium? Vaccine-damaged children are not a rarity, and why do the symptoms mysteriously emerge often at the age of two years after the first round of vaccines?

My views are personal regarding the root causes of neurological disease, but it would be appropriate to seek an expert opinion on running a range of nutritional tests to see where natural treatment could be provided to improve general metabolic function. Certainly, improving dietary intake, replacing vital nutrients, and gently detoxifying through monitored programmes could be of great benefit.

THE IMMUNE SYSTEM

Do you suffer with frequent colds and infections or have been diagnosed with an autoimmune disease?

Poor immune function is a major causative factor in the development of chronic disease.

Boosting your immunity with nutrients and medicinal botanicals can help your white blood cells act more efficiently. The power of your immune system depends on the nutritional power within your diet.

ME—often called chronic fatigue syndrome, presenting with low energy, recurrent sore throats, low-grade fever, muscle and joint pain, intestinal discomfort, emotional distress, depression—can be regarded as an immune dysfunction. These symptoms can last for months or years. The potential root causes—gut, immunity, and liver toxicity—must be investigated. It is not a disease that you catch on the way to work or after an exhausting party. It can be the result of an accumulation of stresses on the body. Getting rundown or living a fast pace of life could be the final factor that tipped the boat.

There is no one answer for restoring immune function. You have to look at all contributing factors—stress, quality of diet and lifestyle, exercise, biochemical genetic inheritance, mental health, frame of mind, environmental challenges, and hormone balance.

Your complex immune system consists of an army of special cells that root out enemies such as viruses, bacteria and fungi that attack the body's defences. Natural killer cells within the immune army can destroy cancerous cells and are often the body's first line of defence.

EFFECTS OF ALCOHOL ON THE BODY

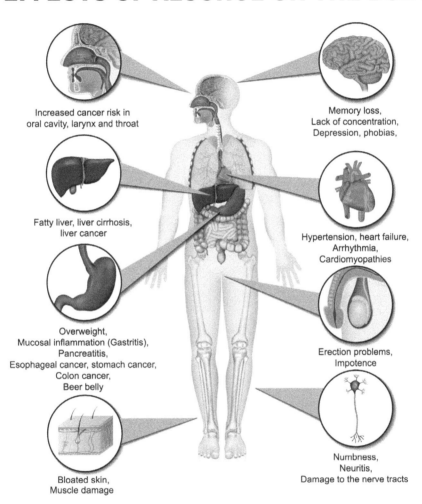

Increased cancer risk in oral cavity, larynx and throat

Fatty liver, liver cirrhosis, liver cancer

Overweight, Mucosal inflammation (Gastritis), Pancreatitis, Esophageal cancer, stomach cancer, Colon cancer, Beer belly

Bloated skin, Muscle damage

Memory loss, Lack of concentration, Depression, phobias,

Hypertension, heart failure, Arrhythmia, Cardiomyopathies

Erection problems, Impotence

Numbness, Neuritis, Damage to the nerve tracts

The immune system is a hugely important, complex, and remarkable tracking army of white blood cells that are constantly on guard, looking to jump into action to protect you from infection and keep you well. This system works within the gut to control pathogens that result from faulty digestion, as well as throughout the body in various areas where teams of white blood cells work in unison to destroy invaders.

The major gland of the immune system—the thymus gland—needs specific support. Nutrients are vital, but spirulina, chlorella and plants with anti-microbial properties boost immune activity and are immune enhancing.

Acid alkaline balance, digestive problems, gut microflora, excessive free radical activity, antioxidant deficiency, leaky gut or poor immune function are some of the potential underlying factors linked to degenerative and inflammatory joint disorders.

Autoimmune disorders that affect connective tissue structures include lupus and ankylosing spondylitis. There are, however, common underlying factors linked to many of these diseases.

Apart from genetic disposition, faulty lifestyle, diet, and weight issues play a major part in poor muscular skeletal health, acting as triggers for autoimmune reactions and degenerative disease. Poor liver function allowing toxic accumulation can often add to the general picture.

THE NERVOUS SYSTEM

You cannot race around in a perpetual state of stress and not expect consequences. During stress, the body, quite sensibly, switches off digestive processes and concentrates on getting its hormones back in balance.

We are all exposed to stresses throughout life. A degree of stress is healthy, and it helps us to keep a balanced metabolism. It is when stress gets out of control that the body can start to suffer physically.

In the alarm stage, the body reacts to acute stress by quickly producing hormones to help mobilise enough energy to deal with the problem. Adrenal insufficiency arises when stress continues in a chronic form and the body tries to adapt to the stress by producing other hormones from the stored energy in the muscles and liver. Eventually, the body weakens as this energy source runs out. Finally, if stress becomes the norm in your life, the body no longer has the energy and reserves to contain it and physical symptoms set in as body systems fail. This results in 'burnout'—adrenal exhaustion and a state of chronic fatigue.

This is now a frequent complaint in modern society and this important root cause of ill health needs urgently addressing.

Dietary cravings and obsessive eating habits are common in modern society, where every dietary wish can be granted. As vital nutrients are depleted, the body hasn't got the wherewithal to withstand relentless ongoing stress.

When unresolved stress escalates, you can become more vulnerable to sickness and disease. There is also pressure on the cardiovascular and digestive systems as the body tries to maintain equilibrium. As the digestive processes switch off under extreme stress, you can very well imagine the disruption to your intestinal tract if stress is a regular part of your life.

STRESS RESPONSE SYSTEM

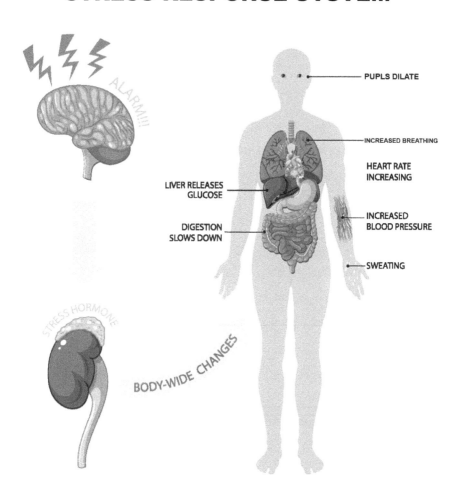

To reduce your fight or flight hormones when they are getting out of control, you need to take steps to combat the source of the stress in your life.

Blood sugar imbalance due to eating sugar, processed carbohydrates, and the frequent use of alcohol or other stimulants stresses the nervous system and causes hormonal havoc.

Depression can result from a disturbed blood sugar balance. This can sap your energy and contribute to mental fog, which can lead to chronic fatigue, anxiety, and many other states of poor health.

Your gut and brain are linked by intricate nerve pathways. What goes on in your gut can profoundly influence your mental state. A direct cause and effect situation. Adequate energy production to manage stress depends on good digestion and absorption of nutrients. If these are lacking or in short supply, then tolerance to stress can be limited.

Stress can be the original causative factor promoting the development of ill health. It also exacerbates existing diagnosed disease and makes recovery a slower process.

Obesity and being overweight

Obesity is defined by having a body fat percentage that is above average.

A healthy body mass index is 18–25%.

The overweight index is 25–30%.

Obesity is over 30%.

An excessive amount of visceral body fat represents an increased risk of disease. It is not only the visible fat but the unseen, invisible fat lining arteries and the heart muscle that increases this risk.

Even being moderately overweight puts a huge strain on body systems and stresses the back, legs, and internal organs. Eventually, mobility can be affected.

Obesity increases the risk of diabetes and blood sugar imbalance. Weight issues reduce the resistance to disease and increase susceptibility to infection. Obesity puts an individual at risk of developing coronary arterial disease and other serious disorders.

Having excess weight to carry around is bound to weaken the body over time and, as one ages, this situation gets worse.

Belly fat on men results in a high risk of degenerative disease, cardiovascular disease, stroke, and dementia. Male abdominal fat is linked to poor liver health.

Exercise, a healthy diet, a positive state of mind and not leading a sedentary way of life are the usual recommendations.

Other cause and effect considerations

Obesity can exacerbate or contribute to muscular skeletal disorders

One of the most important factors in maintaining good skeletal and muscular health is keeping a healthy weight, together with the correct acid alkaline (pH) balance in your cells and tissues. The type of food you eat determines the pH of your tissues and cells. Keeping the body in a slightly alkaline state reduces inflammation and pain. Acidity causes a loss of calcium from your bones and deposits in joints and arteries.

Osteoarthritis, known as a degenerative joint disease, is a wear and tear condition. We all go through many wearing-down processes through life, but the critical point is how well you repair and heal. Do you have sufficient protein in your diet to produce the amino acids that repair your cells and are you overweight?

Are you digesting well enough for the body to absorb nutrients—vitamins A, C and E, and essential fatty acids for cellular repair and lubrication? Do you live a stressful life, creating acidic conditions in your body?

Rheumatoid arthritis is an autoimmune inflammatory condition that affects the entire body, a situation where one's own antibodies attack the joint tissues. Both diseases have some common underlying causes, and which are mainly gut related. If these can be identified and treated, inflammation can be halted, pain reduced, and further degeneration blocked.

Carrying excess weight will exacerbate these conditions. Nutrients have to reach muscle tissue by the bloodstream via the circulatory system. By a similar process, waste material and debris from metabolic function needs eliminating. Cells receive well-absorbed nutrients via the bloodstream, and this process is enhanced by daily exercise and adequate water intake.

Two-way benefits occur when you stretch your limbs as part of daily exercise. By lengthening and then relaxing and contracting the muscles, nutrients are forced into muscles and toxins are forced into the waste disposal side of the lymphatic system. This is designed to shunt the waste into organs that eliminate it—the skin, kidneys, bowels, and lungs.

Zinc and vitamin B6 are required to produce stomach acid, which breaks down protein into the amino acids that the body can use. Within the cells, vitamins B2, B12, folic acid and magnesium are required for protein to enter the energy-making cycle. Once the nutrients enter the cell, vitamins B1, B2, B3, copper and vitamin C complete the process of energy and heat production. So, you can see how vital a nutrient-rich diet is.

PART III

STARTING THE PROCESS OF RECOVERY

Self-help to support and heal the gut

Diet:

- Eat organic food to avoid pesticides/herbicide residues on produce.
- Eat small, well-balanced freshly prepared portions. Never overeat.
- Avoid artificial additives in convenience foods.

Eat regular protein snacks to aid healing. Nuts and seeds are ideal, or wheat-free crackers and plant protein spreads. Later, when healing is complete, eat goat's cheese, as it is more easily digested than cow products.

Increase your intake of protein and fat (coconut can help with the energy production in cells) to improve cellular repair. Avocados are ideal.

Eat plenty of fresh fruit (excluding pineapple, which can irritate the gut lining), as well as vegetables, nuts, seeds, legumes, and wheat-free grains (modern wheat is lacking in nutrients and indigestible due to crossbreeding). Fruit is best combined with oats and nut milk.

Avoid all added sugar, wheat products, strong spices, dairy products, and red meat—they stress the digestive system and irritate the gut. Avoid stimulants, for example strong black tea, coffee, sugar, alcohol, and fizzy drinks.

Drink water between meals, not with meals as this dilutes gastric juices. Eat sea salt for vital nutrients, not table salt. Eat smaller portions under calm conditions to ensure full digestion.

Balance the protein, fat, and carbohydrate in each meal. This ensures that the right vitamins, minerals, and trace elements are available. Chew well, as the carbohydrate-digesting enzyme in saliva starts its first stage of breaking down your food in the mouth.

Eat light protein—eggs and fish regularly and gently steamed vegetables. Avoid salad if you have digestive discomfort. Avocados, cooked carrots, and potatoes are nutritious and nourishing. Cook ancient protein-rich grains, or millet or oats as porridge. Add nuts and seeds to fresh fruit to eat with the porridge. Coconut milk, nut milk or cream can replace cow's milk. Later, goat products can be added.

Having a daily omelette provides the essential amino acids to help repair the gut lining. Rice milk soothes irritation when gastric pain strikes. You need a bland diet with a light protein intake and a healthy balance of essential fatty acids to heal the gut lining.

The soluble fibre in oats, lentils, fruit, and vegetables will ensure that your bowels keep active and healthy, but the insoluble fibre found in the outer husks of whole grains may irritate a sensitive intestinal tract. Choose protein-rich, softer grains such as quinoa, amaranth, and millet, which are nutritious and easy to digest.

If tolerated, eat a mixed green salad with oil dressing before the main meal (avoiding vinegar). A small amount of lemon may be tolerated when mixed with avocado or pumpkin seed oil. Salad contains live enzymes that aid digestion. If salad is not tolerated, eat an avocado and some sprouted seeds (alfalfa or mung bean) with linseed or pumpkin seed oil before your main meal to achieve the same effect.

Supplements to consider:

Gentle plant enzymes can be used with gastric problems (not irritating animal enzymes) (Similase by Nutri Advanced is ideal as they recycle and help the body to produce more enzymes).

Berberine & Grapefruit seed (Nutri Advanced) helps eliminate unhealthy bacteria in the intestinal tract.

Bio Clear (Invivo) is an anti-microbial product that helps cleanse and disinfect the gut.

Quality high-dose multi-vitamin mineral formula (Viridian or Terranova).

Omega 3 and 6 oils EPA/DHA and GLA help nourish and heal the gut.

N-Acetyl-D-Glucosamine (NAG) (Biocare) heals the gut.

Betaine HCl boosts the acid environment of the stomach when low levels of stomach acid are indicated (Biocare). Be cautious of this product if you suffer from gastritis—sandwiching the capsule between food mouthfuls can help, but do not use directly before a meal.

Rezcue, L-Glutamine and zinc carnosine (Thera Nordic) is used to repair the damaged gut lining.

Freeform amino acids (G&G) are the 20 essential amino acids that help tissue renewal.

Beta carotene and vitamin E. Vitamins A and E help heal the gut lining.

Bromelain helps with the digestion of protein in the stomach and clears any undigested matter in the gut. Be cautious with this product if you suffer from gastritis. Pineapple contains this enzyme as an alternative.

B complex, magnesium glycinate and buffered vitamin C in a version that does not irritate the gut lining.

Gamma oryzanol, Marshmallow or Slippery Elm can soothe inflamed tissue (Biocare).

Probiotics—acidophilus are beneficial bacteria that are dominant in the small intestine, where most food digestion and absorption takes place.

Bifido bacteria are dominant in the large bowel. Be cautious if you are suffering from pain, as the lactic acid in acidophilus and fermented food products can irritate your gut.

Tips:

Aloe vera juice (100% organic), potato juice, beetroot or carrot juice have soothing, healing effects and can reduce inflammation. They are alkaline fluids.

L-Glutamine is an amino acid that, together with zinc in a carnosine form, can help restore damaged intestinal lining. Zinc and vitamin B6 are needed for stomach acid production. B vitamins, manganese, magnesium, biotin, copper, iron, and zinc are needed to digest carbohydrates, fat, and protein.

L-Glutamine is the main fuel source for cells in the gut, and it helps restore normal function in the small intestine and can promote healing after surgery or radiation. Normally, the body produces enough glutamine. It is a protein used in healing processes, but in times of extra stress production may be low.

NAG helps to repair the viscous layer of the intestinal lining. This protects the lining from coming into contact with stomach acid and the enzymes that digest your food, as well as the unhealthy microbes that can damage the gut.

GLA is a fatty acid that helps reduce inflammation and protects the intestinal cells from damage from toxins. It has an anti-inflammatory effect.

Probiotics—healthy bacteria to replenish the microflora can be taken when the gut lining is fully healed, and you feel that progress has been made.

I have included some brand names that I use in practice.

Lifestyle:

Avoid all stressful situations that may affect your gut. Get plenty of rest to allow healing. Establish a healthy sleep pattern. Use a botanical essential oil massage after and in a bath as this can aid relaxation.

Tests to consider:

Comprehensive Digestive Stool Analysis with Parasitology

Parasitology, Bacteriology, and Fungal profiles

Allergy and Food Intolerance profiles

Intestinal Permeability assessment

Gastrointestinal Effects profile

Nutritional profile

Self-help to support healthy liver function

Diet:

Eat a balanced, healthy diet that is rich in plant food—beans, fruit, wholegrains, vegetables, nuts, and seeds, plus oily fish. Avoid dairy, wheat, sugar, red meat, and animal fat. Avoid stimulants such as alcohol, coffee, and processed carbohydrates. Do not fry foods and make certain you are using non-hydrogenated cooking oils and healthy fats. Do not use margarine and processed oils that have had their molecular structure changed by chemical processing—these are dangerous, causing free radical damage which harms the body. Olive/avocado oils are best for cooking and use cold pressed natural oils—linseed, hempseed, walnut, and pumpkin oils can be used for dribbling on food.

Drink plenty of water to aid detoxification and especially before bedtime.

Eat less calories each meal. Balance each meal to ensure you eat the correct proportions of healthy carbohydrates, fat, and protein.

Add foods that are beneficial for the liver: apple, artichoke, asparagus, beetroot, chicory, dandelion, celery, carrot, kale, beans, buckwheat, cabbage, endive, garlic, grapes, berries, and cherries. Fennel, lemon, millet, parsley, radish, turnip, walnut, watercress, sunflower seeds, onion, leeks, ginger, grapefruit, and cinnamon are more options.

Avoid detrimental foods: alcohol, animal fat, chocolate, coffee, sugar, fried foods, peanuts, red meat, dairy, modern wheat, and white processed flour products.

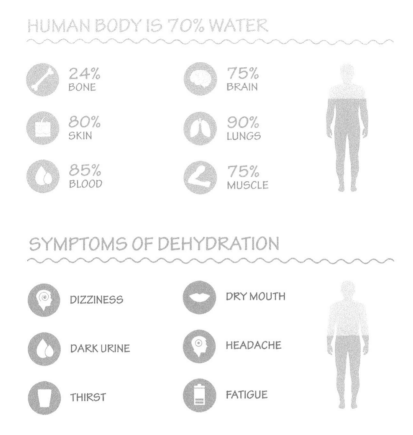

HUMAN BODY IS 70% WATER

24% BONE

75% BRAIN

80% SKIN

90% LUNGS

85% BLOOD

75% MUSCLE

SYMPTOMS OF DEHYDRATION

DIZZINESS

DRY MOUTH

DARK URINE

HEADACHE

THIRST

FATIGUE

Supplements to consider:

Milk Thistle (milk thistle or silymarin can prevent liver damage, help reduce fatty deposits and aid liver regeneration). It also increases bile production and prevents gallstone formation.

Liver detox formulas (G&G).

Multi-vitamin and mineral formula (Terranova).

Sulphur-containing amino acid formula for the detoxification of the liver pathways.

Antioxidants (Terranova) to limit cell damage.

Alpha Lipoic acid as a potent antioxidant.

Phosphatidyl lipid complex.

Magnesium citrate or bisglycinate to aid fat metabolism.

Omega 3 and 6 oils.

Detox formula.

Multi-vitamins and mineral formula (Viridian).

Zinc and B6.

Spirulina (a tonic taken as a smoothie drink).

Antioxidants.

Vitamin C and bioflavonoids.

B complex vitamins in low doses.

Beta carotene.

Tips:

Do not burn food when barbecuing or cooking. Burnt substances cause free radical damage to cells and are carcinogenic.

Repeated exposure to environmental pollutants from your food, water, and the air can overburden the liver, reducing its capacity to clean up your body efficiently. Such an overload has the potential to cause systemic damage to any part of your body. Long-term exposure causes oxidative stress in cells, and they may struggle to absorb nutrients and produce energy. As a result, you may experience chronic fatigue.

Toxic waste lingering in your body resulting from impaired detoxification can cause chronic health problems. In an unhealthy liver, these toxins can migrate to other parts of the body and be stored as fat in the brain, abdomen, and central nervous system. If the liver is unable to clear the toxins due to a lack of nutrients, these will be released into the bloodstream and deposited elsewhere.

The ability of your liver to do this job efficiently determines your state of health and your risk for disease. If you are suffering from poor health, it is vital to avoid chemicals in food and to live a clean lifestyle that helps all your organs support your recovery.

Turmeric and dandelion help support healthy gallbladder and liver function.

Lifestyle:

Take frequent daily exercise in fresh air. Avoid all rich foods. Enjoy plenty of relaxation and rest.

Tests to consider:

Nutritional profile

Amino Acid profile

Fatty Acid profile

Liver Detoxification

Oxidative Stress

Heavy metal toxicity

Comprehensive Digestive Stool Analysis with Parasitology

Other cause and effect considerations

Self-help for neurological conditions

Diet:

Eat a diet that is rich in protein and fat for amino acids and fatty acids.

Avoid all added sugar and stimulants such as strong tea, alcohol, and coffee. Replace with nutritious drinks—warm apple juice, carob powder cocoa with milk, grain, or chicory coffee. Use natural fruit sugars for snacks such as dates, figs, and dried fruit.

Eat whole foods with complex carbohydrates (wholegrains) and avoid white processed flour products.

Basic dietary balance must be improved, and adequate hydration offered as water—often, dehydration can cause extra stress and anxiety. Water also supports healthy detoxification, which is necessary for individuals on medication. Nutrient-rich food is important—processed food is lacking in nutritious elements. Fruit and vegetables, nuts and seeds, legumes, and wheat-free grains, eggs, oily fish, poultry, and meat should be part of your daily diet.

Supplementation must be undertaken only under the guidance of a professional healthcare provider. There are many beneficial foods and supplements that may be inappropriate for certain conditions but may worsen symptoms for people on medication.

Tips:

Research has also shown there can be many benefits following the use of medicinal herbs in terms of alleviating distressing symptoms. A medical professional in tune with functional medicine may be able to guide you through some of the recommendations in this book.

In 1993, Vera Schreibner, PhD, exposed in her book, *100 years of Orthodox Research*, studies showing that vaccines represent a medical assault on the immune system.

Nutritional deficiencies can exacerbate these conditions, as can dehydration and side effects from prescribed drugs.

There is interesting reading for doctors, nutritionists, patients, and carers in a book published in 1996 by Dr Geoffrey Leader MB and Lucille Leader Dip ION titled *Parkinson's Disease—the New Nutritional Handbook*.

Mental and Elemental Nutrients by Carl C Pfeiffer PhD, MD of The Brain Bio Centre, USA contains fascinating reading on the use of nutrients to improve brain activity and improve quality of life for those suffering with neurological disease.

Self-help for improving immunity

Diet:

Eat well-balanced colourful organic food.

Avoid frying and barbecuing foods, as this can generate free radicals and prompt oxidative damage in your cells. Avoid processed food and the regular intake of stimulants that can undermine your immunity by stressing your body. Avoid all sugar as this hormone disruptor suppresses immune function.

Eat adequate protein to support healthy immune function and healthy fats.

Eat fruit and vegetables, as varied and fresh as possible. Eat all colours of the rainbow for antioxidants. Generally, if your immune system in underfunctioning, a higher protein diet including yoghurt rich in lactic acid would be beneficial. Include a good balance of essential fatty acids from oily fish, nuts, and seeds. Eat spices, herbs, onions and garlic, apple cider vinegar and cooking condiments such as juniper berries to disinfect the gut.

Supplements to consider:

Multi-vitamin and mineral formula (Terranova or Viridian).

Multi-antioxidant formula (Terranova).

Echinacea, astragalus and other anti-microbial botanicals listed in *On Guard* or below.

Essential oil of oregano, highly effective for respiratory and digestive infections. Contains potent active ingredients such as thymol and carvacrol.

Olive leaf extract.

Cat's claw.

Vitamin C and bioflavonoids.

Vitamins A, D, and E.

Beta carotene.

B complex vitamins.

Zinc.

Siberian Ginseng for stress.

Essential fatty acids for tissue renewal.

Free form amino acids (G&G) for maintenance of immune cells.

Tips:

Your mind and emotions can affect your immune system. It is well recognised that stress, particularly chronic stress, can suppress immune function. A lack of sleep and late nights also stress the immune system and its ability to function well.

Use herbs with anti-microbial/anti-inflammatory effects:

- Thyme, garlic, onions, turmeric, curcumin, horseradish
- Cloves, cinnamon, chamomile, rosemary, fennel, ginger
- Cardamom, peppermint, nettle, thyme, pau d'Arco, myrrh
- Black elderberry, echinacea, black walnut, goldenseal, berberine
- Artemisia, gentian, oregano, black seed oil (nigella sativa)

Lifestyle:

Fresh air, regular exercise, plenty of rest and a good sleep pattern can regenerate immune cells.

Drink plenty of water between meals and use other healthy fluids such as herbal teas and vegetable juices.

Tests to consider:

Immune Antibody tests

Antioxidant profile

Nutritional tests

Toxic Elements profile

Mucosal Immune Reactivity Screen

Gut Immunology profile

Oxidative Stress

Other cause and effect considerations

Poor immunity and detoxification can be linked to cancer

A dreaded word, but many cancers have been overcome by dealing with potential underlying root causes.

Exposure to toxins in the workplace, to pesticides, herbicides sprays or by smoking cigarettes and vaping are well-known carcinogenic triggers. Synthetic hormones such as HRT increase the average cancer risk, and these are just a few of the risk factors.

If these factors are coupled with an incorrect diet, damaging lifestyle, nutrient deficiencies, poor detoxification, and immune dysfunction, then cellular renewal can be adversely affected. Toxin-free fuel is required by the body to build healthy new cells.

Building up immune strength to reverse the growth of cancer cells with nutritional medicine and phytotherapy is the way forward. Many studies have shown it possible to treat cancer with natural protocols that boost the body's self-healing processes and reabsorb tumours. View Chris Woollams' website www.canceractive.com.

Treat the body, not the cancer. The latter is the body's natural response to detox cells, clear out infections, replace missing nutrients, and renew old cells. This process just needs extra support.

Proteolytic enzymes can unmask cancer cells and disintegrate the protein fibrin—these are designed to clear up debris in the human body.

Conventional cancer treatments are invasive and destructive, but embarking down this route is a very personal choice. At least, one should follow all the best natural drug-free advice on supporting a healthy body. Natural approaches can have amazing success rates, but these figures are supressed by the pharmaceutical giants that profit from chemotherapy. The success rates for cancer have hardly altered over the decades of debilitating treatments and billions spent on research. But the pharmaceutical companies call the shots. It is illegal to quote success or advertise in favour of natural therapies. Chemotherapy makes billions.

Self-help for cancer

Diet:

Eat only organic.

Avoid all processed foods, alcohol, sugar, animal fat, red meat, dairy products, coffee (this is a roasted product), modern wheat, and excess carbohydrates. All grain carbohydrates should be in a complex, nutrient-rich whole form (as in ancient grains) and not processed white flour products.

There are numerous diets currently in use by cancer patients, depending on the type of cancer and other factors. Sugar feeds cancer, so a carbohydrate-rich diet is not recommended. Likewise, a high-protein diet is not ideal due to the acidic internal environment that it creates. Moderation is the answer—eating an organic, well-balanced, and freshly prepared nutrient-rich diet.

Generally, a diet rich in fruit and vegetables can help to deliver as many nutrients as possible, especially if it contains lean protein, beans, and lentils. Go grain free unless protein-rich ancient grains such as amaranth, quinoa and millet or dinkel are used. Modern wheat is hybridised; it is hard to digest and lacks vital nutrients. Focus on eating sulphur-containing foods such as cauliflower, onions, and garlic which provide liver support.

Legume pasta is fine, but not wheat pasta. Go for wild rice but not processed rice.

Beneficial omega oils include walnut, avocado, pumpkin, and linseed. Quark and yoghurt can aid immunity by increasing glutathione production. Glutathione is an amino acid used by the liver for detoxification.

Avoid all environmental toxins where possible. These include food additives, body care products containing harmful chemicals, or cleaning product vapours that can be absorbed through the skin or nose.

Supplements to consider:

Black seed oil (Nigella Sativa).

Cat's claw.

Garlic.

Essiac tea.

Berberine (Hadley Wood).

Artemisia.

Medicinal mushrooms (G&G).

Antioxidants with Resveratrol.

Multi-vitamin and mineral formula (Terranova).

B complex.

Selenium and vitamin E.

Zinc.

Vitamin A.

Bioflavonoids and vitamin C.

There are many medicinal plants—too many to list here—that have been shown to exhibit anti-mutagenic/metastatic activity (also known as anti-tumour effects). Essiac is well worth investigating.

Clinics that favour natural treatment for cancer have had very promising results. But, as natural treatments are not supported and are recognised as controversial, cancer sufferers are not given this alternative information and are left with few choices other than accepting treatment that is aggressive—poisoning, surgically removing or radiating their tumours. However, these choices of improving every system in your body are out there. Treatments that do not cut-burn-destroy and, sometimes, damage healthy cells.

The bottom line is—give patients well-studied choices of treatment and support them if they refuse conventional oncology treatment to go down the natural route.

Tips:

There are wonderful cancer clinics worldwide fighting to heal their patients—healing without doing harm, as Hippocrates taught. There is much scientific research on the nutritional approach to cancer. Refer to the Resources section to Further Reading.

Consulting with a professional functional medicine practitioner experienced in integrative oncology would allow you to focus on, or combine, various conventional and/or alternative approaches. It is your body—you should not be forced, by threat of early death, into treatment you are not in tune with. There are many options open to you.

Try to explore every avenue by doing well-documented research and choose what is right for you.

Lifestyle:

Stress-free, including meditation, yoga, and relaxation classes. Fresh air and outdoor pursuits. A healthy sleep pattern and activities that involve concentrating the mind.

Tests to consider:

Nutritional

Oxidative Stress

Free Radical profile

Liver Detoxification

Comprehensive Digestive Stool Analysis

GI Effects

Self-help to alleviate stress

Diet:

Eat a diet high in protein and fat and avoid simple carbohydrates in the form of white flour products, sugar, and alcohol. Eating double the amount of protein to carbohydrates at meals helps to balance your blood sugar level and stabilise stress.

Avoid all other stimulants and eat regular, well-balanced meals with healthy snacks. Hydrating well can balance your blood sugar levels– **it takes 2 molecules of water to metabolise 1 molecule of glucose.**

By increasing your intake of protein and fat, you avoid initiating an insulin response. These foods also help you to balance blood sugar levels to combat the stress. They are bodybuilding, repairing foods and take longer to digest than the energy foods—carbohydrates. Protein and fats calm and reduce stress levels, helping you to return your body to a state of relaxation—in the same process, optimising brain function to help focus and clear thinking.

Well-balanced nutritious meals need to be eaten three times a day, making sure that breakfast is packed full of the nutrients the body requires to supply the day's energy needs. Birchermuesli would fit the bill to start the day—containing yoghurt, coconut, fresh fruit, salad, nuts, seeds, and complex wheat-free protein-rich wholegrains, all mixed together in a bowl, adding 100% organic fruit juice to reach the right consistency. Eat vegetables, salad, protein-rich grains, nuts and seeds, egg, fish, meat, and dairy.

Deficiency signs of protein include depression, mental health problems, stress, nervous disorders, and hormonal problems.

Essential fatty acids (EFAs) help you control stress by:

- Regulating nerve transmission
- Controlling blood pressure in the eyes, joints, and blood vessels
- Improving muscle reflexes and lubrication of all body tissues
- Maintaining the health of cell membranes
- Influencing immune and anti-inflammatory responses
- Helping maintain healthy heart function
- Supporting mental health and reducing stress

Food sources of essential fatty acids:

Organic nuts and seeds—linseed (high in omega 3), sunflower, pumpkin, sesame, hemp, evening primrose and borage oils.

Walnuts (high in omega 3) and oily fish—mackerel, herring, salmon, and sardines.

Keeping your fatty acids in balance can support every body system and help to reverse disease and heal the body.

Investigating the health of your intestinal tract is the number one consideration when dealing with stress. Initially, you should check whether these essential fatty acids are part of your diet and then whether you are converting them correctly.

Supplements to consider:

B complex vitamins—in particular, pantothenic acid vitamin B5 for the adrenal glands.

Zinc and B6 for blood sugar balance, healthy adrenal glands, and digestion.

Bioflavonoids.

Ashwagandha.

Siberian Ginseng relief for long-term chronic stress, a general tonic that is also immune boosting.

Rutin, which strengthens the blood vessels.

St John's Wort—a natural mood booster.

Vitamin C.

Omega 3 and 6 oils, which nourish the nerve cells.

Digestive enzymes with HCL.

Multi-vitamin and mineral formula (Terranova or Viridian).

Liver detox formula with milk thistle (G&G).

Tips:

Calcium and magnesium taken before bed can help you to relax. Herbal teas have a beneficial calming effect.

Kava, valerian, lemon balm, rhodiola, passiflora and chamomile aid sleep. This effect is cancelled if you continue drinking stimulatory drinks.

Drink smoothies with chlorella and spirulina in either the morning or evening for a nutritious rich intake of micro- and macro-elements.

Increase your intake of potassium-rich foods such as potatoes, bananas, and other fruit. Eat protein at each meal. Eat snacks regularly—ideally nuts and seeds, or cheese and fresh fruit.

A fatty acid imbalance can be linked not only to stress but other conditions such as arthritis, depression, hormonal disturbances, blood sugar dysfunction and cardiovascular disease. Deficiencies can affect any area of the body, as these essential fats are part of the structure of cells.

It has also been established that the sufferers of skin conditions such as eczema and psoriasis experience an impaired conversion of EFAs. This highlights the need for nutrients for the conversion process.

Shingles, scabies, and other skin rashes are usually the result of viral, bacterial, or fungal overgrowth together with nutritional deficiencies and/or an underfunctioning immune system.

EMF—Electromagnetic field exposure is producing many zombie-like individuals that are in a permanent state of stress that promotes mental health problems. As the world sinks into a sea of technical devices that give little time for relaxation, matters can only get worse in the future. If the body has no time to relax, little time to digest food and is deficient in the nutrients needed to repair body cells, chronic poor health is just around the corner.

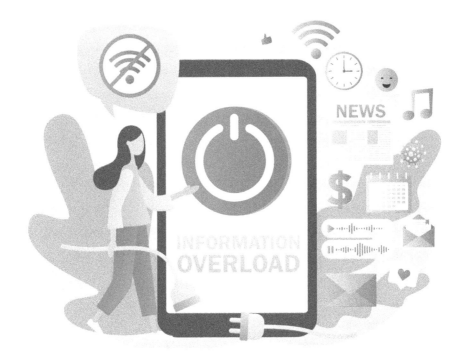

In the 1970s and 80s, Dr Carl Pfeiffer at The Brain Bio Centre in New Jersey in the USA used nutritional therapies to overcome psychological disorders from depression, stress, and anxiety to schizophrenia. He showed that when a proper biochemical balance was achieved through dietary changes and supplementation, the body returned to a state of good mental and physical health. He believed that good nutrition was the way to prevent disease. He found that excess copper in the body had been found to be a brain stimulant. Copper is essential for maintaining life, but in excess it can be toxic. The use of the 'Pill' and HRT can cause a toxic copper overload. When copper is high, it competes with zinc—and zinc is vital, as it participates in dozens of enzyme functions and is a vital brain trace element. High levels of copper reduce the absorption of zinc. Dr Pfeiffer used zinc in therapy with patients with excess copper and had amazing results.

The detection of adrenal insufficiency that contributes to stress disorders can be seen in **Hair Mineral Analysis**, an analytical test that measures the mineral content of your hair. This reflects the mineral content of your tissues over a 3-month period.

Lifestyle:

Understand your hormones and natural body clock. Live in tune with your body and don't challenge your body systems by eating a poor diet or leading an unhealthy lifestyle. Everything in moderation.

Take gentle exercise. Enjoy meditation if this is your thing—or yoga, swimming and cycling out in the fresh air. Get out in the sunshine without sunscreen to soak up vitamin D (but not in the heat of the day and not for prolonged periods).

Tests to consider:

Adrenocortex Stress profile

Nutritional profile

Amino Acid profile

Fatty Acid profile

Hormonal profiles

Comprehensive Digestive Stool Analysis

Self-help to reduce weight

Diet:

Reduce your calorie intake, avoid saturated animal fat, and balance your blood sugar levels. Alcohol is a major culprit contributing to weight increase.

Reduce your intake of starchy and fatty foods.

Increase your intake of fresh fruit, salad and vegetables, wholegrains, nuts, and seeds. Eat light protein, oily fish, and occasional eggs.

After sustained improvement is seen, you can add light lean protein such as poultry and lamb. Drink water between meals only to aid digestion and last thing at night to aid detoxification, but never with meals. This dilutes your stomach acid.

Avoid all sugar and grains except millet, oats, quinoa, and amaranth. Eat smaller, well-balanced meals. Reduce your intake of starchy foods—potatoes, rice, pasta—and sweet fruits such as pineapple and grapes. Berries are healthy and contain less natural sugar.

Eat more protein and healthy plant fat to lose weight. Limit carbohydrates and eat fibre-rich foods, both soluble (fruit, legumes, and vegetables) and insoluble (grains). Beans, peas, lentils, and chickpeas are healthy options to meat and provide the necessary fibre for the bowels when combined with wheat-free high-protein grains.

Fresh produce contains live enzymes that help you digest your food more efficiently. Chilled, fresh products in supermarkets have had their enzymes destroyed by the temperature changes during transportation and supermarket display. This is more or less 'dead food' and readily decomposes—an example of which is carrots going black soon after purchase. Carrots traditionally keep for weeks and months when stored correctly. But supermarkets thrive on a quick turnover so the quality of produce suffers and, as a result of us eating it, we may experience digestive problems. Buying at open markets is the best practice.

Medium chain triglycerides can increase thermogenesis (burning off fat). The main sources are coconut oil and low-fat dairy products. Coconut oil is lower in calories than olive oil or avocado oil and can be used as a readily available energy source when cooking.

Supplements to consider:

C0Q10 to help oxygenation and circulation.

Multi-vitamin mineral formula (Terranova).

B complex vitamins to optimise the metabolic rate (Viridian).

Zinc and B6 for stomach acid and insulin production.

Vitamin C and bioflavonoids speed up a slow metabolism and support healthy glandular function.

Choline and inositol help the body burn fat.

Chromium and vitamin B3 help stabilise carbohydrate metabolism.

Kelp to increase metabolic rate and thyroid activity.

Lecithin (sunflower) to emulsify dietary fat.

Tips:

Metabolic nutrition

Eat fat to burn fat. This might sound a load of nonsense, but certain foods we eat are converted very quickly into heat. This is called thermogenesis. Overweight individuals produce less heat during thermogenesis; nevertheless, it is still beneficial to eat thermogenic foods as they can stimulate an underfunctioning metabolic rate, providing adrenalin which raises body temperature.

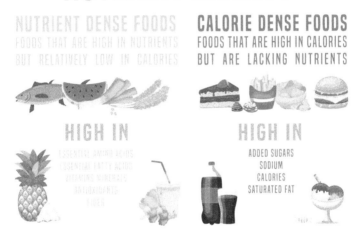

NUTRIENT DENSITY

NUTRIENT DENSE FOODS
FOODS THAT ARE HIGH IN NUTRIENTS
BUT RELATIVELY LOW IN CALORIES

CALORIE DENSE FOODS
FOODS THAT ARE HIGH IN CALORIES
BUT ARE LACKING NUTRIENTS

HIGH IN
ESSENTIAL AMINO ACIDS
ESSENTIAL FATTY ACIDS
VITAMINS MINERALS
ANTIOXIDANTS
FIBER

HIGH IN
ADDED SUGARS
SODIUM
CALORIES
SATURATED FAT

Thermogenic foods include apple cider vinegar, mustard, cinnamon, vinegar, green tea, hot spices, whey protein powder, coconut fat, ginger, and black pepper.

Cold water can also help kick-start your metabolism to warm up your body.

Calorie counting doesn't work. It is the quality of your calories, not the quantity of your calories, which gives you the biggest success.

We all house an individual genetically programmed metabolism. Foods that have a positive effect on one person may have the opposite effect on another.

When stress is high and your batteries are run down, it is only natural to grab the first sugary goody available. Energy loss, dizziness and sleepiness are signs you have run out of glucose. But this bad habit is taking you down a slippery pathway to ill health. If too many carbohydrates are eaten, more than the body can use for energy, then the excess will be stored in the brown fat cells.

The only types of food that can turn this sorry state of affairs around are proteins and fats. No insulin is produced when eating fat and protein, so these foods can be used for repair and maintenance, with the added benefit of making you feel full and satisfied with a calm gut and mind.

Stimulants and 'pick-me-ups' have a similar effect. Especially coffee, as one can easily become addicted to caffeine and other chemicals in coffee beans. It will be hard to wean yourself off this central nervous system stimulant, but it is unhealthy to drink coffee regularly. It contributes to the development of cardiovascular disease, interferes with sleep patterns, disrupts hormones, causes anxiety and restlessness, and results in a hyped-up nervous system, and an increase in heart rate.

Increasing the amount of protein in the diet helps to stabilise blood sugar levels. It gives a feeling of satiety after meals. The result of this eating pattern is that your body will be stimulated to burn off its stores of fat.

Protein and reasonable amounts of healthy fat, which the body needs for cell repair, do not cause an increase in weight.

Protein deficiency can cause weight increase as the body eats far too many calories to control its fluctuating blood sugar levels.

In the USA, where high-fat meals are consumed, the picture may be different. Weight increase could be equally due to an excess of fat or carbohydrate.

Indigenous tribes around the world who eat unprocessed foods and mainly carbohydrates generally are lithe and lean. Their carbohydrate source is not processed and laden with chemicals that, in the Western world, cause toxic conditions in cells.

Only dietary changes can reverse a fatty liver. Despite being an organ that can regenerate readily, if the liver is seriously diseased, repair may not be possible. Look for the warning signs. If your body fat index is high and you are obviously overweight, with your shape showing dangerous signs of abdominal fat, there needs to be an action plan.

Good fats/bad fats

All cell walls contain both fats and protein. Your brain is over 60% fat, so the fats you eat need to be healthy ones.

Fats keep hunger at bay, and they take three times as long to digest as carbohydrates and are an efficient way to store energy.

Essential fatty acids increase the metabolic rate in the body and help burn off fat, as already mentioned. Additionally, they help to avoid the build-up of unhealthy hard, saturated animal fats.

Good fats include butter, nuts and seeds, and plant oils such as olive, flaxseed, hempseed, pumpkin seed, walnut, avocado, oily fish, and coconut fat. Other healthy oils can be found in blackcurrant seeds, borage, evening primrose oil, safflower, and sunflower, providing that these oils are cold pressed and unprocessed. Healthy oils should not be heated (excluding olive and avocado oil).

Essential fats lubricate your cells and keep the electrical activity of your heartbeat in sequence.

Bad fats include processed, modified, hydrogenated, or partially hydrogenated oils. They function as saturated fats in the body and can be responsible for free radical damage, as the natural healthy molecular structure has been damaged by processing. Listed as trans fats, they are toxic and damaging.

Margarines and other spreads are all processed. The body cannot use these damaged oils.

Freeform amino acids are predigested, and well-absorbed spirulina contains vital nutrients and usable protein, thereby stabilising your blood sugar levels.

Various amino acids stop sugar cravings.

Lifestyle:

Do stretching exercises daily and engage in outdoor activities such as walking, cycling, and jogging for at least an hour daily. Try to keep active throughout the day with only short periods for relaxation.

Skin brushing can be of benefit to increase circulation.

Tests to consider:

Organic Acid profile

Cardiovascular profile

Fatty Acid profile

Comprehensive Digestive Stool Analysis

Amino Acid profile

Cardio Check

Hormonal profiles

Metabolic profile

Liver Detoxification profile

Oxidative Stress

An assessment should be made as to whether insulin resistance is contributing to the build-up of fatty tissue. How the body handles fat, carbohydrates and protein is an important issue.

Self-help for muscular skeletal health problems

Diet:

Eat lighter forms of protein—seafood, fish, poultry, and eggs. Avoid all sugar, wheat, dairy, red meat, and stimulants such as strong tea, coffee, and alcohol, all of which are acid forming and promote inflammation. Avoid all processed and hydrogenated cooking fats. Use avocado oil/olive oil for cooking.

Eat an alkaline-rich diet with plenty of greens, fruit, and vegetables. Reduce your intake of saturated animal fat. Increase your intake of anti-inflammatory foods: nuts, seeds, plant fats (avocado and coconut), walnuts, and linseeds which contain omega 3 oils, all of which fight inflammation.

Increase your intake of magnesium-rich foods (greens) and reduce your calcium intake.

INFLAMMATORY FOODS

FRIED FOODS

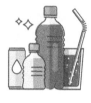

SODAS

REFINED CARBS

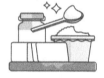

LARD

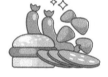

PROCESSED MEATS

Eat smaller portions at mealtimes with regular, healthy snacks such as fruit, nuts, and seeds to help balance blood sugar levels. This reduces stress. Chew well and take time for meals. Keep hydrated.

Avoid weight increase and, if obese, deal with measures to burn off stored fat.

Supplements to consider:

A multi-vitamin and mineral product (Viridian).

Joint care treatment (Taka Turmeric) for inflammation.

Joint and muscle ease treatment (Armour Natural) for inflammation.

Joint massage oil (Viridian) for inflammation and pain relief.

EPA/DHA omega 3 fatty acids from fish oil for anti-inflammatory support.

Antioxidant multi-formula (Terranova or Viridian).

B vitamin complex.

Vitamins A, D, E, K and C.

A quality multi-vitamin and mineral formula (Terranova or Viridian).

Full spectrum freeform amino acids for tissue repair. Provides all 20 amino acids used by the body in a predigested form that can be assimilated after exercise (G&G brand).

Digestive enzymes and HCL (Viridian or Pure Encapsulation).

Magnesium glycinate or sulphate.

Liver detox formula (G&G).

Spirulina and split-cell chlorella for trace elements and detoxification.

Quercetin, Boswellia, Curcumin and Glucosamine sulphate.

Zinc Methionine.

Tips:

Minor aches and pains may be linked to deficiencies of magnesium, an imbalance between calcium and magnesium due to too much calcium present in the diet, or from you not eating enough magnesium-rich foods such as dark green leafy vegetables, whole grains, nuts, and seeds.

Chlorophyll—the green pigment in plants such as greens and algae—contains a lot of magnesium. Calcium contracts your muscles and magnesium has the opposite effect of relaxing muscles. Deficiencies of the essential fatty acids that help lubricate tissues can promote aches and pains, as well as liver and gut disorders. Always pay attention to gut health and optimise function wherever you can.

The wrong diet high in trans fats, saturated animal fats and processed cooking oils can result in pro-inflammatory responses if the conversion of fats is compromised.

The correct diet contains healthy unprocessed fats, resulting in an anti-inflammatory response. This is very significant if you are suffering from inflammatory disease—you can see here that reversing symptoms may require significant major changes in diet.

Eating an alkaline-forming diet will help control inflammation. Try to eat mostly plant foods—fresh fruit, vegetables and salad, beans, and grains, in particular ones that are rich in magnesium.

Drink plenty of water to flush out toxins, as well as lubricate and alkalise tissues.

Nuts, seeds, avocado and oily fish have anti-inflammatory effects and help with lubrication and the repair of new cells. Linseeds and walnuts contain omega 3 fatty acids and are particularly healthy.

Lifestyle:

Avoid stress. Get plenty of restorative sleep.

Gentle, regular stretching exercises will tone and strengthen your muscles. This is ideal after a warm bath with relaxing oils or Epsom salts to detoxify tissues. Avoid challenging, hard exercise that overly stresses the body. Take regular, gentle oxygenating exercise such as walking, swimming (reduces stress on the joints), yoga if tolerated and cycling.

There are many healing massage oils that you can use:

- Frankincense and lavender oils to massage the muscles
- Thyme oil can be inhaled to help reduce inflammation and pain
- Arnica oil helps relieve pain
- Rosemary oil aids circulation
- Rose oil to soften and lubricate the skin

Always use a carrier oil to dilute.

I recommend Weleda products for the bath milks and massage oils.

Tests to consider:

Nutritional profile

Metabolomics and Nutritional test

Inflammatory Markers

Comprehensive Digestive Stool Analysis

Metabolic Analysis

Essential and Metabolic Fatty Acid test

Osteoporosis assessment

Self-help for skin complaints

To keep your skin healthy, drinking an adequate amount of water is the foremost requirement. Water carries nutrients to the cells and is the medium for flushing out toxins. It also lubricates.

Natural skincare products are vital, and they should be chemical-free and pure.

Weleda/Laverna/Sante products are excellent.

If the skin is damaged, it requires amino acids from proteins for repair, together with essential fatty acids from oily fish, nuts, seeds, and plant foods. Dry skin and other skin disorders can be a sign of essential fatty acid (EFA) deficiency, or deficiency of the nutrients needed to metabolise and convert fats. This conversion process is dependent on adequate levels of vitamin B6, biotin, zinc, and magnesium. The fat you consume has to be emulsified by lecithin and broken down into small units called micelles, which are a form that can be absorbed.

Sulphur-containing foods such as onions, garlic, cauliflower, and brussels contain the sulphur-containing amino acids L-Methionine and L-Cysteine. These are essential for the structural growth and maintenance of your hair, nails, and skin.

Milk thistle (silymarin) is a useful herb that nourishes the liver and reduces cell proliferation and inflammation. This herb helps to heal psoriasis, a skin disorder that is linked to liver problems.

Sulphur can also fight bacterial infection on the surface of cells and can more generally help tone up the skin.

Certain chemicals, burnt food, alcohol, and eating trans fats (processed oils) can block the enzyme processes that convert healthy fats from food into micelles—and, further on, into prostaglandins, a type of hormone that regulates inflammation.

Self-help for eye conditions

Diet:

Eat plenty of rainbow foods, a varied diet containing all the colours that nature provides. These yellow, red, and pink/red pigments—lutein, lycopene and astaxanthin—keep the eyes healthy. Eat red, black, and blue berries, especially bilberries that contain other pigments.

These improve circulation and help nutrients reach the eyes. Eat plenty of dark greens rich in chlorophyll. Eat mineral-rich foods. Eat foods rich in beta carotene, which converts to vitamin A. This protects the internal tissues of the eyes. Eat a varied balance of essential fatty acids from seeds, nuts, plant oils, coconut, and oily fish.

Reduce your intake of animal fat and dairy products. Avoid damaging stimulants—sugar, coffee, alcohol, and processed carbohydrates such as wheat. The overconsumption of these foods produces too much glucose, which gets into the circulation and damage the eyes.

Supplements to consider:

Omega 3 and 6 essential fatty acids.

Evening Primrose oil (Viridian).

Sulphur-containing amino acids (Biocare) for tissue repair.

Multi-vitamin and mineral formula (Terranova or Viridian).

Magnesium Taurate (Taurine is required to keep your eyes healthy) (Biocare).

Lutein, Lycopene and Astaxanthin—carotenoid pigments to control free radical damage (Viridian).

Vitamin E and selenium.

Gingko biloba for circulation.

Antioxidant formula (Terranova).

Eyebright—a herb to improve eye health.

Tips:

Splash your face with cold water after washing—this helps blood flow. Gently massage around the eyes. Avoid dust and irritating substances such as barbecue smoke.

Lifestyle:

Take daily exercise to oxygenate your tissues. Drink water regularly between meals to lubricate and to help bring nutrients to the eye tissue.

Tests to consider:

Nutritional profile

Fatty Acid profile

Antioxidant profile

Comprehensive Digestive Stool Analysis

Self-help for heart disease

Diet:

Avoid all acid-forming food and habits—smoking, alcohol, saturated animal fat, dairy, sugar, coffee, and red meat. Drink plenty of water to hydrate your tissues and help the absorption of nutrients. In rare cases, surgery has been avoided after initiating water therapy as it hydrates and dilates the blood vessels—this alone can bring great benefit, together with exercise and dietary changes. I have witnessed this in my own clinic.

Your diet should be mostly plant based. Eat plenty of colourful fruit and vegetables full of plant chemicals and antioxidants that support the heart—complex wholegrains, healthy fats from oily fish, seeds, beans, seafood and occasional eggs or lean poultry. Avoid heavy meals. Many heart attacks have occurred after a large, fatty meal.

Replace coffee—a stimulant—with chicory that aids liver and digestive function.

Eat sea salt for vital nutrients, not table salt.

Supplements to consider:

Vitamin C and the amino acid L-Lysine can help restore health, reabsorb atherosclerotic plaque, and promote healthy circulation. Vitamin C is anti-inflammatory and helps thin the blood.

CoQ10 is an oxygenator and antioxidant (G&G or Nutri Advanced).

L-Carnitine (G&G) is an amino acid that is beneficial for the heart.

Lecithin (not soya but sunflower) emulsifies the fat from your diet, ensuring that it is broken down effectively for correct absorption.

Phosphatidyl choline improves fat metabolism.

Pycnogenol (Pure Encapsulations) is an antioxidant that protects cells from oxidative damage.

Potassium is required for heart function.

Superoxide dismutase (SOD) is a powerful antioxidant (G&G).

Lycopene and Lutein pigments (Viridian) are powerful antioxidants. These are among the yellow and red pigments found in food.

Antioxidant and bioflavonoid complexes (Terranova).

Multi-vitamin mineral heart formula (Terranova).

B vitamins, particularly vitamin B3 which can help dilate arteries.

Homocysteine to lower complex H Factors (Higher Nature).

Vitamin E and selenium.

Omega 3 fish oils and essential fatty acids to provide omega 3 for anti-inflammatory support.

Proteolytic enzymes—Serrazyme (Good Health Naturally) or Serrapeptase (Now Foods) for scavenging plaque.

Vitamins A, zinc, and magnesium Taurate.

Garlic to thin the blood.

Tips:

Proteolytic enzymes such as Serrazyme/Serrapeptase can be taken to help reduce arterial plaque. Magnesium supports muscular action, and essential fatty acids help to decrease platelet build-up and the tendency towards thrombosis. Homocysteine is a toxic substance produced in the body by a biochemical process called methylation. Raised blood levels are linked to a higher risk of developing blocked arteries. Adequate B vitamins, zinc and Betaine for the methylation process prevent this production.

Antioxidants that keep your cells healthy and stop fats from oxidising are vital to help halt the process of further deterioration.

B vitamins, magnesium, antioxidants vitamins A, C and E, selenium, and zinc are required to help reverse heart disease. Vitamin C acts also as an anti-inflammatory agent. Taurine, an amino acid, has a favourable effect on the heart muscle.

Suboptimal levels of any vitamins and minerals can increase the risk of disease.

Lifestyle:

Measured and monitored exercise is necessary for serious disease, otherwise regular gentle activities such as walking, stretching, and swimming, which are designed to oxygenate and regenerate the circulatory system, are vital. You need to revitalise your body.

Avoid stress. Get plenty of relaxation and establish a restful sleep pattern. If you suffer from heart disease, you will need a radical overhaul of your diet and lifestyle—looking at every angle to see how to improve and support the cardiovascular system and produce a happy heart.

Tests to consider:

Amino Acid profile

Comprehensive Cardiovascular profile

Homocysteine

Oxidative Stress profile

Fatty Acid profile

Nutritional profile

Antioxidant profile

Comprehensive Digestive Stool Analysis and Parasitology

These tests analyse insulin and glucose tolerance, fatty acid balance, comprehensive blood lipid status, nutrient balance, fibrinogen affecting blood coagulation, C-Reactive Protein (an inflammatory marker), and Homocysteine, a marker for increased cardiovascular risk, and other genetic risk analytes.

Many of these markers are important indicators for individuals who may not otherwise appear to be at risk and who do not currently suffer from heart disease.

With modern advances in research, acting on the early warning signs can significantly change the progression and direction of the disease.

Self-help for infertility

Diet:

Avoid alcohol and other stimulants, as well as sugar and wheat. Do not drink dark black tea. Tannic acid causes a loss of alkaline minerals. Darjeeling/oolong or green tea is a better option.

Eat a protein-rich organic balanced diet with healthy fats and oils. Increase your intake of nutrient-rich foods such as fruit, vegetables, salad, nuts, seeds, and legumes.

Eat wholefoods and organic natural produce to avoid toxins.

Eat regular meals and keep hydrated to improve nutrient balance in cells.

Eat zinc-rich foods—nuts, seeds, kale, mushrooms, eggs, beans, seafood, grains, dairy, meat, and avocado.

Supplements to consider:

Zinc and vitamin B6 (for female hormonal balance and improved male sperm count and motility).

A quality multi-vitamin mineral designed for pre-conceptual care (Natural Health Practice, Marilyn Glanville's products).

Hormonal support (Natural Health Practice).

L-Arginine (for sperm health).

Essential fatty acids omega 3 and 6.

Freeform amino acids (G&G).

B complex.

Tips:

Copper levels in women on the pill or using the coil are often elevated. As copper and zinc work in tandem in the body, this excess copper competes with the absorption of zinc. Zinc is crucial for both partners and there should be more zinc than copper in the cells. Many factors can affect fertility, but foremost are vitamin and mineral deficiencies. Zinc, arginine—an amino acid—and vitamin B6 are all required for a healthy sperm count.

The regular intake of alcohol can reduce zinc levels. If you are trying for a baby, the health of both partners is equally important.

Dietary toxins and heavy metals can disturb the balance of nutrients in cells.

Low protein in the diet, or the poor metabolism of protein due to low stomach acid and zinc/vitamin B6 deficiency, can affect fertility. Hormones are made out of protein.

For successful conception and a healthy pregnancy, you need to improve your overall health, and that of your partner. Avoid stimulants and avoid smoking.

A pre-conceptual programme for six months prior to conceiving can improve your chances of producing a healthy baby.

A list of pre-conceptual care practitioners can be found in the Resource section at the end of this book.

The way forward is to identify and remove toxins, check for genito-urinary and intestinal infections, assess your nutritional balance, identify nutritional deficiencies, treat any digestive or malabsorption problems, and improve your biochemical balance. Eat organic food and drink filter water—tap water can contain synthetic hormones, heavy metals, nitrates, pesticides, and chlorine, all of which are damaging to the human body.

Lifestyle:

Avoid late nights and establish a good sleep pattern. Take regular gentle exercise in the fresh air. Avoid stress.

Tests to consider:

Hormonal tests

Nutritional profiles

Amino Acid profile

Fatty Acid profile

Toxic Elements test

Comprehensive Digestive Stool Analysis with Parasitology

PART IV

YOUR ACTION PLAN SUMMARY

Eat regular meals consisting of organic, well-balanced food.

Modern diets, even organic ones, are not always 100% rich with nutrients. Many factors are linked to the production of food: the climate, the state of the soil, the purity of water, the atmosphere, harvesting, packaging, transport—and there are many linked to the state of the environment in general. But the very best you can do for your health is to eat organic produce—this will protect you in this polluted world.

The first step to good health is having the knowledge to build a healthy balanced meal.

This should contain as many as possible of the necessary nutrients that the body needs daily for growth, repair and energy needs in cells. Shopping can be easy once you know the rules.

The second step to good health is eating a nutritious breakfast.

A fortified, super nutritious bowl of goodness:

Breakfast is the most important meal of the day. A well-balanced mix of wheat-free, unprocessed whole grains, nuts, seeds, fresh colourful fruit, dried fruit, and sugar-free yogurt provides you with many vital nutrients to supply energy for the day ahead.

Nutrients improve concentration, stimulate brain activity, balance blood sugar levels, and boost metabolic function.

Birchermuesli, as it is known today, comes in many forms, all adapted versions of the original Dr Bircher Benner recipe in Switzerland. He formulated a breakfast mix of grains, chopped apple, nuts, seeds, and yogurt to heal the sick patients in his clinic (1867–1939).

Experiment each day with different sun-ripened, if possible, organic fruits, fruit juice, muesli grains, coconut, chopped dates, figs, nuts, and seeds, combined in one bowl with dairy or nut milk options. The mixture should be moist and creamy.

Add also: organic split-cell chlorella, spirulina, and barley grass powders.

Hempseed powder.

Organic flaxseed oil.

Organic protein powder (whey or pea/rice plant protein).

A dash of lemon juice.

Organic raw cocoa nibs.

Compare this nutritious mix to a breakfast of toast and sugared jam. The former with a balance of complex (whole) carbohydrate, protein, and healthy fats—takes hours to digest and provides all the energy you need for the day. The latter—purely processed simple carbohydrate is digested and metabolised quickly, leaving you struggling to get through the morning without a snack to boost your blood sugar levels.

Eat a rainbow diet and a variety of food to ensure a good variety of nutrients.

Starting with macro-elements, you should know how to balance your protein and fat intake, which are both body-building foods, with carbohydrates, which are energy-producing foods. This is an important part of good nutrition. Consider the types of protein, fat, and carbohydrate that you will eat.

There are four basic nutrients vital for our existence, namely water and the macro-elements of carbohydrate, protein, and fat. Within the macro-elements, we find the micro-elements, which are vitamins, minerals, amino acids, and trace elements. These are the nutrients that are absolutely necessary for good health and the optimal functioning of all body systems. There are dozens of nutrients we need to eat on a daily basis, so each meal needs to be nutritionally balanced for your body to function well.

The human body contains approximately 70% water. This bathes our cells, regulates our body temperature, provides the fluidity of our blood, and improves the elasticity of the blood vessels together with fats. Water is essential for the detoxification processes in the liver and aids in the elimination of waste material in the intestinal tract.

If you become dehydrated, signs of this can occur an hour before the event, when you can suffer in many ways—constipation, low energy, mood changes, headaches, migraine, fevers, tight dry skin or dry, prickly eyes. The list is endless where water is concerned. You may be unaware of most of this happening until symptoms develop. Party the night away, eat a lot of unhealthy food, drink alcohol and forget to drink water, then you may regret your actions.

The main dietary culprits are strong black tea, strong coffee, alcohol, and sugar. The latter can contribute to fluid loss in the body by changing the acid/alkaline balance in cells. Tea in particular is highly diuretic. The elderly suffer particularly from fluid loss and offering herbal teas instead of black tea in elderly people's homes would be beneficial for health. In moderation, the body can tolerate these stimulants, but you need to compensate for the effects with regular water intake. Plain water is best because, if any other flavouring is added, this reduces the time it takes for the fluid to filter through the kidneys.

Drinking water with meals dilutes the stomach acid. Your stomach acid is precisely that, an acid. It needs to be acidic to digest protein. Diluting it is not a good practice. In time, digestive problems can develop in individuals that have low stomach acid production to start with. The time to hydrate is between meals and at night.

Trying to run your body on a slice of toast with sugary jam and a cup of strong coffee that dehydrates is not a good idea if you want to keep healthy. The end result, sooner or later, will be poor health or disease.

Healthy food choice

Put as many colours of the rainbow on your plate as possible: fresh fruit, vegetables, and salads. Be sure to include starchy portions of potatoes, wholegrain pasta, rice, beans, and legumes, as well as nuts, seeds, and oils.

Eat a fibre-rich diet; this forms the basis of healthy stools and provides food for the growth of beneficial bacteria.

Digestion works well with a high-fibre diet and fibre protects against many major diseases. Constipation and haemorrhoids can be a sign that the body is lacking in fibre. Medication will not help. But changing your habits will.

Health problems are reversible and treatable providing the root causes are dealt with. You cannot patch up a body with drugs whilst ignoring the basic underlying root causes of disease.

The food you eat provides the fuel that runs your body.

When it comes down to it, 96% of your body is made up of chemical elements—carbon, hydrogen, oxygen, and nitrogen. All of these are present in the macro-elements of your diet—the fundamental dietary building blocks of carbohydrate, protein, and fat.

There are numerous biochemical enzyme pathways involved in the processes that break down carbohydrates, protein, and fat into small nutrients—these are the micro-elements that can be used by the body for energy, repair, and the growth of all cells.

Carbohydrates are metabolised into energy—every cell needs energy to function. Protein and fat, along with a few minerals, are the elemental building blocks used for renewing and maintaining the health of new cells. Vitamins are absolutely essential for health as they regulate the thousands of chemical reactions that keep us healthy and alive.

You are, quite literally, what you eat, digest, and absorb.

All metabolic and biochemical pathways in the human body are dependent on the dozens of nutrients present in your food, but they have to reach the cells, and this means good digestion and absorption. Healthy eating is not just a fad. It can represent the difference between health and disease, living or just existing.

It has been estimated that the average diet is rich in the macro-elements of protein, fat and carbohydrates, but lacking in many micronutrients such as zinc, magnesium, vitamin B complex, and vitamins A, C and E. The very fuel necessary for good health.

Change old habits

We live in a fast-paced, fast-food society. It's all there for the taking—supermarkets brimming with readymade meals, sugary snacks, buns, cakes, and goodies to grab when time is short. It requires willpower to go straight to the healthy organic section to buy your food, but it is worth it—your body is worth it. It is the only one you have, and it needs to last you for a long time.

It is forgivable when needs be; you may be needing food, any food—quick! Often, instant food right from the shelf. I have sometimes been in this situation. But this is hardly the type of fuel that sustains health in the long term. Even then, you should seek out the healthier options of fast food and definitely go for what is sugar-free. Dates, nuts, and figs are a healthy snack alternative, or bananas.

Western societies are actually suffering from malnutrition—specifically, not from a lack of calories, but a lack of many of the vital nutrients that are required for good health. Malnutrition inhibits the body's natural defence systems which protect us from common degenerative diseases such as cancer and heart disease.

Modern diets are so low in nutrients that many people are not in the best state of health. They may actually find the odd niggly symptoms of poor health to be absolutely normal. After all, they seem to be part of daily living. The price to pay for enjoying all of the fast food available.

The human body is a wonderful work of art that works intricately well given the right conditions. It will always strive to keep your cells happy and your metabolism running smoothly. Unfortunately, our bodies mildly protest over a long period of time and are very accommodating when offered substandard fuel. You can become complacent and not recognise the need to act. After all, it looks appetising, has wonderful marketing blurbs on the packet…it can't be that bad.

During these times, you may feel twinges of discomfort, feel unwell or become under the weather. These are the first signs that your cells are not happy as you munch away on sugary snacks. It takes time for nutrient deficiencies and symptoms to develop. As the matter becomes serious, panic sets in. How can food be the culprit? How could such a simple thing as diet be the root cause of serious diseases?

Everything has a beginning. A point where changes take place in the cells of the body, a point where nutritional deficiencies develop, damage to the cell structure occurs and systems start to fail.

Some individuals have an increased need for nutrients—the pregnant for development of the embryo, the young for body growth and development, the elderly for body maintenance and repair, the sick for convalescence and healing, athletes for energy output and recovery, and smokers and drinkers for detoxification and cell protection.

Improve your digestion

Minor symptoms of poor health can be cleared up simply by making positive changes to your diet. Adding nutritional supplementation to correct deficiencies acts as an insurance policy against developing deficiencies in the future. If your life is always stressful, I recommend taking general supplementation on a daily basis.

Serious diagnosed disease where medication is being used requires collaboration with a suitably qualified practitioner. They will monitor dietary changes and guide you through the complex supplement programmes that must be compatible with your medication.

The goal should be to investigate the underlying causes of your condition through test procedures and to finally discontinue medication. If it is not possible for you to discontinue drugs, an effort should be made to follow all basic guidelines in this book, correcting deficiencies, rebalancing body systems, improving diet and making sure your lifestyle is healthy. Refer also to my book *Chronic Digestive Disorders*.

Using supplementation requires expert advice if you are seriously ill. A practitioner will run tests and prescribe supplements appropriate to the test results. They will use the correct doses for your individual biochemistry. Some nutrients are water soluble and rarely become toxic if overdosed. However, fat-soluble vitamins such as vitamins A, D, E and K need careful monitoring as they are stored in the fatty tissue and can be very toxic in inappropriate doses.

If you choose to do so, or already have to remain on prescribed medication for the rest of your life, the least you can do is eat the sort of diet that supports the liver detoxification pathways and take general supplementation that replaces the lost nutrients that will occur from medication use. The general health of your whole body cannot be ignored just because you need permanent medication. Any action, however small, is better than no action at all, and you will soon feel the benefit of feeding your body correctly with renewed energy and an improved state of health.

Basic tips:

Use herbs in cooking, but avoid strong, irritating hot spices.

Avoid fizzy drinks and food additives.

Eat organic produce and nutrient-rich foods. Read labels for added sugar.

Nourish your gut lining with foods that heal (check the digestion and gut section).

Take plant-based digestive enzymes to help break down your food if required.

If required, use hydrochloride HCL to help digest your protein meals.

Take a quality multi-vitamin mineral product daily.

Take a quality probiotic to help re-colonise with healthy gut bacteria.

Take the time to chew well. Do not eat under stressful conditions.

Eat more protein and healthy fats to improve your digestive function and combat stress.

Look at labels, and check both quality and composition. Cheap products can sometimes contain harmful ingredients.

I recommend the following brands of supplementation: Viridian, Invivo, Nutri Advanced, G&G, and Terranova. I have no vested interest in these companies.

Good health is influenced by your individual biochemistry and inherited genes. But you do have a choice when it comes to steering your body in a healthy direction. The expression of your inherited genes depends on your diet and lifestyle, as you do not necessarily inherit the disorders that run in your family. Choose food that is compatible with your individual metabolism and the type of healthy diet that you feel well on.

You may think, how can I do that? Well, if you generally feel well on a daily basis, you are eating the right food balance. Get to know your body and it will soon tell you when your diet needs adjusting.

Clear up any infections—Further advice is in my book *On Guard*.

If you are sick and unwell and not on medication, the following steps can be taken:

Take medicinal herbs at the recommended dose on the bottles.

These herbs have a profound positive effect on bacterial, fungal, or viral infections and often nourish the body at the same time.

Use plant medicinal massage oils to support your supplementation therapy.

If you are under medical care and taking prescribed medication:

Seek a functional medicine practitioner in the medical field who is favourable to these approaches.

If you have been diagnosed with a medical condition and are currently under treatment, taking all of the basic recommended dietary and lifestyle steps to nourish and heal your body is relevant to achieving recovery.

When the body remains sick within, disease will continue to flourish.

Drugs should never be stopped and replaced with supplements—the latter should only be taken under expert care of a professional.

Detoxify your body:

Exercise regularly and practise deep breathing and stretching exercises.

Avoid chemical cleaning products.

Use natural chemical-free body care products.

Use biocompatible dental materials.

Eat organic wholefoods. Check all labels for nasty, damaging chemicals.

Drink plenty of pure water. Use a filter if in doubt.

Eat foods that aid liver and gallbladder function.

Increase your protein intake to support your liver detoxification pathways.

Take a quality multi-vitamin and mineral detox product daily. After improvement take a multi- vitamin mineral product as an insurance policy to maintain good health.

Soak in detoxifying essential oil baths.

Use massage oils to detox and destress.

Deal with stress issues.

Seek professional help if appropriate. Do yoga, meditation, and exercise.

Slow down your pace of life. Reduce your screen time.

Pace your space when under pressure.

Manage weight.

Excess weight stresses the body and puts you at an even higher risk of serious disease.

Metabolic slimming can help in this area. Eat thermogenic foods that will help you burn off fat.

Every step you can make in taking control of your body will aid recovery.

Look upon food as your medicine and your lifestyle as your wellness centre. Your body is designed to heal itself.

It is a misconception that life can only be enjoyed with alcohol, junk food and sugary snacks.

Life is best enjoyed when you feel positive, full of energy and 100% fit.

This only comes from well-balanced food and a healthy lifestyle.

Exercise regularly outdoors

You need fresh air, quality water and daily activity outdoors. Avoid obsessive electronic gadget use. Mental stress in modern society is a real threat, with most individuals unable to do without their smart phones. It is an unnatural dependence and needs monitoring and planned usage to allow you the freedom of life that existed a few years back. It is a necessary part of modern life, but addictive all the same.

We cannot slow progress in the world, but what you can do is avoid a toxic environment as much as possible. Limit your screen time, enjoy a varied, healthy outdoor life, and an organic diet. Recognise your body's limits and don't overdo things. It will take time out of your life to recover.

No matter how unwell you feel, the body can rejuvenate and help to build a new you.

Find a professionally trained functional medicine practitioner to guide you through the vast array of biochemical tests available and to monitor treatment and progress. Serious disease sufferers will need professional care.

PREVENTION IS ALWAYS BETTER THAN CURE

It is impossible to be completely 100% pure in a world full of damaging substances, but the measures outlined in this book will help reduce risk and keep you fit and healthy. Having a positive attitude, enjoying an engrossing hobby, and seeking harmony with nature will help both body and mind to be at peace with the world.

Nutritional therapy is a preventative form of medicine. It supports the body within by boosting the function of all body systems with nutrients to aid healing and prevent disease.

In Andrew Saul's excellent book, *The Orthomolecular Treatment of Chronic Disease* (listed in the further reading section), 65 leading experts for therapeutic and preventative medicine show how, for the last 80 years, large therapeutic doses of vitamins have been successfully shown to cure and reverse serious chronic illness.

OPTIMUM NUTRITION MEANS:

- **Protection from infection and disease**
- **Resistance to stress**
- **Support for maintaining robust health**
- **Improved mental function and clarity of mind**
- **Healthy digestion and absorption of nutrients**
- **Maintained energy levels and stamina under pressure**
- **Restorative sleep patterns**
- **A feeling of good health and well-being**

Food can offer specific support as: natural laxatives, anticoagulants, painkillers, beta blockers, antioxidants, insulin regulators, tranquillisers, antidepressants, blood fat balancers, decongestants, vasodilators, expectorants, anti-inflammatories, and antibiotics.

Supplements can replace many drugs, but I strongly advise you to seek the advice of a healthcare professional to guide you through the correct steps and monitor your progress.

Give your health 100% attention if you seek good health, and follow all the guidelines in this book to experience how it is to feel really well again and full of energy. Then take one day out and eat unhealthy meals—sugar, stimulants, and processed food. Observe the results. The 'before and after' feeling should be enough to point you again in the right direction.

The quality of your life is ultimately in your hands.

I wish you well on your journey to better health.

REVERSE SICKNESS AND ENJOY GOOD HEALTH AGAIN

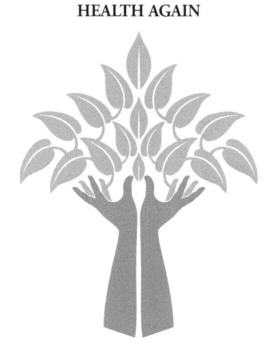

FURTHER READING

What to Eat if you have Cancer by Daniella Chase and Maureen Keane. ISBN 0-8092-3261-8. Published by Contemporary Books 1996

Great News on Cancer in the 21st century by Steven Ranson. ISBN 1-904015-07-7. Published by Credence Publications UK 2002

The Cancer Handbook – What's really working by Lynne McTaggart. (What Doctors Don't Tell You Publication) Published 1997

Say No to Cancer by Patrick Holford. ISBN 0749919511. Reprinted by Piatkus 2001

The Optimum Nutrition Bible by Patrick Holford. ISBN 978-0-7499-2552-9. Published by Piatkus 2004

Mental and Elemental Nutrients by Carl Pfeiffer. ISBN 0-87983-114-6. Published by Keats 1975

Uninformed Consent by Hal Huggins, D. D. S and Thomas Levy. ISBN 1-57174-117-8. Published by Hampton Roads Publishing Company 1999

Cure Tooth Decay – Heal and Prevent Cavities with Nutrition by Ramiel Nagel. ISBN 13:978-0-9820213-0-9. Published by Golden Child Publishing 2012

Trace Elements and other Essential Nutrients by Dr David Watts. ISBN 1-885676-15-8. Published by Watts 1997

Thorsons Guide to Amino Acids by Leon Chaitow. ISBN 072252492 7. Published by Burns & Smith Ltd 1991

Heart Disease – Heart Disease can be Prevented and Reversed Using Clinically Proven Alternative Therapies by Burton Goldberg. ISBN 1-887299-10-6. Published by Alternative Medicine Digest 1997

An Alternative Medicine Guide to Cancer by Burton Goldberg, John Diamond MD and Lee Cowden, MD. ISBN 1-887299-01-7. Published by Future Medicine Publishing Inc. 1997

Turning a Blind Eye by Robert Redfern. Published by Eyesight Action UK 2004

Parkinson's Disease The New Nutritional Handbook by Dr G. Leader MB. and Lucille Leader Dip ION. ISBN 0 9526056 1 9. Printed by The Bath Press 1996

Nutrition and Mental Illness – an Orthomolecular Approach to Balancing Body Chemistry by Carl Pfeiffer, PhD. ISBN 0-89281-226-5. Published by Healing Arts Press 1987

Eat Drink and be Merry – Basic Principles of Illness Prevention and Treatment using Nutritional and Environmental Medicine by Tuula Tuormaa. ISBN 1 898941 52 1. Published by Country Books 2001

Vaccination by Vera Scheibner, PhD. ISBN 0 646 15124 X. Printed by Mc Pherson's Printing Group Australia 1993

The Vaccination Bible by Lynn McTaggart. A 'What Doctors don't Tell You Publication' 1997

Vaccinations and Immunisation: Dangers, Delusions and Alternatives by Leon Chaitow. ISBN 0-85207-191-4. Published by C. W. Daniel Company Ltd 1987

Syndrome X – The Complete Nutritional Program to Prevent and Reverse Insulin Resistance by Jack Challem, Burton Berkson, MD and Melissa Diane Smith. ISBN 0-471-35835-5. Printed by Wiley 2000

An Alternative to Psychiatry by Tuula Tuormaa. ISBN 0 863325831. Published by The Book Guild 1991

The Orthomolecular Treatment of Chronic Disease by Andrew Saul, M.S., PhD. ISBN -10: 1591203708. Published by Basic Health Publications, Inc. 2014. Website www.doctoryourself.com

Dirty Medicine by Martin Walker. ISBN 0 9519646 07. Published by Slingshot Publications 1993

Confessions of a Medical Heretic by Robert Mendelsohn, MD. ISBN 0-8082-4131-5. Published by Contemporary Books 1979

What Your Doctor Didn't Learn in Medical School by Stuart Berger, MD. ISBN 0-380-70319-X. Published by Avon Mooks 1988

How to Live Longer by Vernon Coleman. ISBN 1 898947 24-4. Published by European Medical Journal Publishing House 2001

Gaynor J Greber

The Mind Gut Connection by Emeran Mayer. ISBN 9780062376589. Published by Harper Wave 2018

Modern Medicine for Modern Times by Adonis Maiquez, MD, ISBN-13 978-1515-260233. Published independently 2015 www.Miami-Institute.com (The Functional Medicine Handbook to prevent and Treat Diseases at their Root Cause).

Functional Medicine, The New Standard by Kevin Hoffarth, MD and Charlie Hoffarth et al. ISBN 979-6104-0430-1. Published independently 2020

In-depth medical research What Doctor's Don't Tell You Journal/Magazine.

Latest information on Complementary and Alternative Medicine on all health issues.

https://www.wddty.com

RESOURCES

The Institute for Optimum Nutrition

Ambassador House

Paradise Road

Richmond TW9 1SQ

Tel: 0044 20 8614 7800

Website: www.ion.ac.uk

There is a list of UK practitioners available on their website, some of whom practise functional medicine.

The Institute for Functional Medicine

505 S.336th St Suite 600

Federal Way

WA G8003

Tel: 1.800228 0622

General enquiries: 1.800 228 0622

Email: info@ifn.org

Website: www.ifm.org

There is a worldwide practitioner list on their website.

Mineral Check

Bull Cottage

Lenham Heath Road

Lenham Heath

Maidstone

Kent TN17 2BP

Tel: 0044 1622 850 500

Email: mineralcheck@mineralcheck.com

Website: www.mineralcheck.com

LABORATORIES

Regenerus Labs

Redhill Aerodrome

Aero 14

Kings Mill Lane

Redhill RH1 5SJ

Tel: 0044 203750 0870

Website: www.regeneruslabs.com

USA

Genova Diagnostics

Asheville NORTH Carolina

P.O. Box 3229 Asheville NC

Tel: 28862-3220

Website: www.gdx.net

UK

Genova Diagnostics

46-50 Combe Road

New Malden KT3 4OF. UK

Tel: 0044 208 336 7750

Website: www.gdx.net

Biolab Medical Unit

Stone House

9 Weymouth Street

London W1W 6DB

Tel: 0207 636 5959

Website: www.biolab.co.uk

Pre-conceptual care practitioners

www.forsight-preconcerption.org.uk

Index

Milton Keynes UK
Ingram Content Group UK Ltd.
UKHW020158241023
431186UK00010B/187